ADVANCE PRAISE FOR
TALES FROM THE PAGER CHRONICLES

"This wonderful collection of stories captures both the miraculous and the prosaic work of nursing. These stories remind us of the intimate and profound work of the nursing profession. In addition to amazing stories, Patrice Rancour gives us insight into what it's like for patients, families, doctors, nurses, and other health care professionals to face the challenge of the end of a life."

—Betty R. Ferrell, PhD, RN, FAAN
Research Scientist, City of Hope

Tales from the Pager Chronicles is a moving book—and a call to action. The many dramatic scenarios presented by Patrice Rancour confirm the importance and urgency of the need for palliative care services to be available in every acute-care hospital. The drama, the exasperation, and the crisis management could be avoided as a result of proactive palliative care management, thereby creating the dignified quality of living each and every one of us so desperately want under these circumstances."

—Judy Lentz, RN, MSN, NHA
CEO, The Alliance for Excellence in
Hospice and Palliative Nursing

"Anyone who has experienced one of these many human crises knows how helpful it is to have a guide and companion along on the journey. However, if one is fortunate enough to have a skilled guide like Patrice Rancour, who is informed by the intellect and empowered by competent caring, then one has been more than lucky. One has been blessed."

—Grayce M. Sills, PhD, RN, FAAN
Ohio State University

"This is a 'tell-it-like-it-is' book that gets to the raw emotions that we deal with daily—and hourly—in busy hospitals. Rancour has used patients' stories to bring to us the pain and joy of life—and death. She is a talented nurse and writer. The book will be enormously helpful to people going through cancer.

—Jimmie C. Holland, MD
Memorial Sloan-Kettering Cancer Center

BOOKS PUBLISHED BY THE HONOR SOCIETY OF NURSING, SIGMA THETA TAU INTERNATIONAL

Tales From the Pager Chronicles, Rancour, 2008.

The Nurse's Etiquette Advantage: How Professional Etiquette Can Advance Your Nursing Career, Pagana, 2008.

Johns Hopkins Nursing Evidence-Based Practice Model and Guidelines, Newhouse, Dearholt, Poe, Pugh, and White, 2007.

Nursing Without Borders: Values, Wisdom, Success Markers, Weinstein and Brooks, 2007.

Synergy: The Unique Relationship Between Nurses and Patients, Curley, 2007.

Conversations With Leaders: Frank Talk From Nurses (and Others) on the Front Lines of Leadership, Hansen-Turton, Sherman, and Ferguson, 2007.

Pivotal Moments in Nursing: Leaders Who Changed the Path of a Profession, Houser and Player, 2004 (Volume I) and 2007 (Volume II).

Shared Legacy, Shared Vision: The W.K. Kellogg Foundation and the Nursing Profession, Lynaugh, Smith, Grace, Sena, de Villalobos, and Hlalele, 2007.

Daily Miracles: Stories and Practices of Humanity and Excellence in Health Care, Briskin and Boller, 2006.

A Daybook for Nurse Leaders and Mentors, Sigma Theta Tau International, 2006.

When Parents Say No: Religious and Cultural Influences on Pediatric Healthcare Treatment, Linnard-Palmer, 2006.

Healthy Places, Healthy People: A Handbook for Culturally Competent Community Nursing Practice, Dreher, Shapiro, and Asselin, 2006.

The HeART of Nursing: Expressions of Creative Art in Nursing, Second Edition, Wendler, 2005.

Reflecting on 30 Years of Nursing Leadership: 1975-2005, Donley, 2005.

Technological Competency as Caring in Nursing, Locsin, 2005.

Making a Difference: Stories from the Point of Care, Volume 1, Hudacek, 2005.

A Daybook for Nurses: Making a Difference Each Day, Hudacek, 2004.

Making a Difference: Stories from the Point of Care, Volume 2, Hudacek, 2004.

Building and Managing a Career in Nursing: Strategies for Advancing Your Career, Miller, 2003.

Collaboration for the Promotion of Nursing, Briggs, Merk, and Mitchell, 2003.

Ordinary People, Extraordinary Lives: The Stories of Nurses, Smeltzer and Vlasses, 2003.

Stories of Family Caregiving: Reconsideration of Theory, Literature, and Life, Poirier and Ayres, 2002.

As We See Ourselves: Jewish Women in Nursing, Benson, 2001.

Cadet Nurse Stories: The Call for and Response of Women During World War II, Perry and Robinson, 2001.

Creating Responsive Solutions to Healthcare Change, McCullough, 2001.

The Language of Nursing Theory and Metatheory, King and Fawcett, 1997.

For more information and to order these books from the Honor Society of Nursing, Sigma Theta Tau International, visit the honor society's Web site at www.nursingsociety.org/publications, or go to www.nursingknowledge.org/stti/books, the Web site of Nursing Knowledge International, the honor society's sales and distribution division. Or, call 1.888.NKI.4.YOU (U.S. and Canada) or +1.317.634.8171 (Outside U.S. and Canada).

TALES FROM
THE PAGER CHRONICLES

PATRICE RANCOUR, MS, RN, CS

Sigma Theta Tau International
Honor Society of Nursing®

Sigma Theta Tau International

Editor-in-Chief: Jeff Burnham
Acquisitions Editor: Cynthia Saver, RN, MS
Development Editor: Carla Hall
Copy Editor: Nicole Sholly

Cover Design by: Commercial Artisan, Indianapolis, IN, USA
Interior Design and Page Composition by: Rebecca Harmon

Printed in the United States of America
Printing and Binding by Edwards Brothers

Sigma Theta Tau International
550 West North Street
Indianapolis, IN 46202

Visit our Web site at www.nursingknowledge.org/STTI/books for more
information on our books.
ISBN-10: 1-930538-72-3
ISBN-13: 978-1-930538-72-6
Library of Congress Cataloging-in-Publication Data

Library of Congress Cataloging-in-Publication Data

Rancour, Patrice, 1951-
  Tales from the pager chronicles / Patrice Rancour.
      p. ; cm.
  ISBN 978-1-930538-72-6
  1. Cancer--Nursing. 2. Nurse and patient. 3. Nursing--Psychological
aspects. I. Sigma Theta Tau International. II. Title.
  [DNLM: 1. Oncologic Nursing--Personal Narratives. 2. Nurse-
Patient Relations--Personal Narratives. 3. Nurses--psychology--Personal
Narratives. WY 156 R185t 2008]
  RC266.R36 2008
  616.99'40231--dc22
                                                        2008027579

First Printing
2008

AUTHOR NOTE
Due to the nature of my work, confidentiality is paramount. All names used in the telling of this story are fictitious. Often, circumstances have been intermingled to give composite illustrations of clinical experiences taken from my years of work with life-threatened individuals and their families. While portraits herein are representative, individual privacy has been protected. If any incidents described in this book seem familiar to the reader, it is because these experiences, while unique to each individual, are not unusual.

DEDICATION

I would like to thank Professor Emeritus Dr. Grayce Sills, Ohio State University College of Nursing, for her wonderful network of connections through which I ultimately found myself at Cynthia Saver's door at Sigma Theta Tau International. Thank you, Cindy, for "getting it." I want to thank all of those editors out there who kindly provided me with extremely favorable feedback, but politely declined to publish my manuscript because they didn't know quite what to do with it.

But mostly, I would like to thank the legion of people who allowed me entrée into the most intimate moments of their lives, those patients and their families, who permitted me into the nightmare world of life-threatening illness, just by sheer virtue of the fact that I did have the letters, "RN," behind my name on my name tag. How humbling. And also, how illuminating to be on the receiving end of so many teachings in conscious living and conscious dying. There are not so many work paths that actually provide one with the fodder of how to live a life consciously, but certainly, nursing is one of them. Most people really don't know that much about what nurses do until they need us. And then, it is our privilege to serve.

From a fellow pilgrim on the path, I thank all of you who serve as my teachers. I can only hope I receive all the lessons.

ABOUT THE AUTHOR

Patrice Rancour, MS, RN, CS, has been in the health care field for 35 years as a clinician, educator, and consultant. She received both her undergraduate and graduate degrees from Ohio State University. As a psychiatric/mental health clinical nurse specialist, she has authored 40 papers and has presented at numerous conferences and symposiums. Her primary areas of interest include working with life-threatened individuals and their families, complementary and alternative therapies, spirituality and healing, end-of-life care, and grief and loss issues. She continues to maintain a private practice in addition to her current position working with Ohio State University's Faculty/Staff Wellness Program providing worksite wellness services to university employees. All things being equal, when she isn't working, the author would rather be wandering the shoreline of a certain barrier island off the coast of Georgia.

TABLE OF CONTENTS

FOREWORD

Playing off the old maxim, "the medium is the message," a counter saying developed over the years in relation to nurses. It goes something like, *"The medium is silence and the message is not heard."* This refers to the fact that nurses frequently talk amongst themselves but seldom write or speak about their experiences to those outside the profession. Essentially, they preach only to the choir. In the 1990s, Suzanne Gordon, a New England-based journalist, cast her eye to the nursing profession. Both an advocate and a provocateur, Gordon has exhorted nurses to find and use their voices (Buresh & Gordon, 2006). Patrice Rancour heard that call and, with this book, has officially found her voice.

The work you are about to read offers a richly textured portrait of the work life of a nurse. It is an exquisite exploration into the area sometimes referred to as "explicating the hyphen," that term so blithely inferred when we use the hyphen to describe the roles and functions of positions in direct relationship to one another—nurse-patient, physician-nurse, and so on.

It is in this interior region that deals with the essence of what occurs in relationships where Rancour's voice is at its best. She articulates in beautifully crafted language the complex nature of the interplay in those relationships. We come to know the depth of her intellectual understanding of what is going on with the "other" as well as with herself. The reader comes to feel the empathic awareness of the "other" through her casual yet lovely prose. We come to marvel at the well of compassion that fuels her spirit when the fatigue and weariness of the day intrudes on the work. It is at this level that the non-nurse reader can apprehend the awe-inspiring nature of nurse work. Anyone who has experienced one of these many human crises knows how helpful it is to have a guide and companion along on the journey. However, if one is fortunate enough to have a skilled guide, informed by the intellect and empowered by competent caring, then one has been more than lucky. One has been blessed.

It is my hope that nurses and others will find in these pages the tender and truthful voice of a nurse who has embraced the work of nursing as the profession of relationships. It is said that professions do just that: They "profess" to do something the public cannot do. Or, they do it better than the public can. Rancour tells us that nursing is the profession of relationships, and it is through these thoughtfully bound relationships that we are aided in transitions and facilitated in processing change. Nursing is often portrayed as a caring profession. Certainly this book demonstrates that very well. What is also clear is that underpinning the work is an intellectual understanding of the processes of health and illness. This work is coupled with the creative capacity for empathy and compassion and is bound by an ethical understanding of the existential nature of all human dilemmas.

Personally, it was sometimes painfully difficult to keep reading. The book brought home to me memories of my own loved one's experiences in the intensive care unit. The memories that were aroused in me were still difficult for me to deal with, but in these pages there was also healing and comfort.

So for the reader, colleague or stranger, may you find a voice here that resonates as true, that resonates with a deeper understanding of the profession of relationships—the profession that is called *nursing*.

—Grayce Sills, RN, PhD, FAAN
Professor Emeritus
Ohio State Univeristy

INTRODUCTION

The work of nursing is often hard to bear, which is why it is not for everyone. Being given a socially sanctioned entrée into the warts-and-all shadows of human lives is, as they say, not for the squeamish or faint of heart. But for those with an eagerness to explore the very human realms of conscious living and conscious dying, the work of nursing expands into high art, a true gift to the practitioner. Where else does one get paid for learning how to live—and for that matter, die—on such a conscious plane?

Why write this book? On a very personal level, my contact with the people in these stories filled me up so much that I felt the need to pour them out or I would overflow. Nurses are affected by the people we take care of. It is an error in judgment to believe otherwise. Long after the last time I met with each of these individuals, their gifts continue to pour out of me in ways I never anticipated. An old adage has it that while the learning is in the hearing, the healing is in the telling. The metaphor of the wounded healer must be an apt one for me, as the writing about what my patients shared with me has helped heal those broken places left in me by their loss. (Those places that Ernest Hemingway assured us are made stronger afterward.) Some believe that people come into our lives for a reason, a season, or a lifetime. I guess these unsuspecting folks came into my life for the long haul. I so longed to share what I had learned from the presence of my patients that *Tales* just seemed to organically breathe its way into existence.

One of the occupational hazards of health care work is that it comes at you fast. The idea of being catapulted throughout a day by the call of a pager is readily understood by anyone who has ever worn one. The pressure of being able to cut to the chase quickly when the sheer volume of needs is threatening to swallow one alive is a very real phenomenon, and I wished to convey that clearly in the book. The notion of "pager urgency" when working with cancer patients becomes a critical experience in the reading of the stories. This ultimately became the literary device I chose to use to propel the story line. Emergencies, by their very nature, preclude the opportunity to research the best approach to a situation. The pressing priorities become carving out "enough" time to spend with people who desperately deserve it and then prepare to move on to the next crisis avalanching behind the current one. There is almost never time to contemplate the most ideal solution for every new problem. And so, one of the most palpable features of this narrative is the pressure to be able to tap dance just as fast as possible, always thinking fast on my feet. In the end, it is a trial by fire, often forged in concert with the people being served.

The audiences I wanted to reach are multiple and varied. If you are someone who has a serious illness or who loves someone who has a serious illness, I would like you to read this book as a manifesto of hope. While not everything is "fixed" in what you are experiencing, not everything is "broken" either. I would like you to connect with those unbroken parts, breathe some life into them, and expand them into every inch of your true self. I would like you to remember that you are more than your body, that, indeed, you are a spiritual being on a human path rather than the other way around.

If you are a health care provider, I would like you to read this book as a manifesto of hope. I would like you to focus on everything that you accomplish in a day and not what you were unable to accomplish. I would like you to reconnect to the energy that gives meaning to your work, so that work becomes the prayer you send out into the world. By prayer, I mean to suggest that it is the very real manifestation of your life's purpose.

If you are a professional health care student, I would like you to read this book as a manifesto of hope. You, like the rest of us, are a work in progress. Become mindful of all of us who come into your life for a reason, a season, or a lifetime. For we are all sent into each other's lives as living, breathing teachings.

And if you are someone who does not fall into any of the audiences above, I would like you to read this book as a manifesto of hope.

As a fellow pilgrim on the path, I wanted to "show," not "tell," stories about illness, care-giving, what it means to be alive, and what it means to face the prospect of not being so. (I offer discussion questions at the end of the book for those interested in exploring these and other topics more in depth.) Not all of us have the advantage of working with people facing such quandaries, so hold your true self larger. Remember that you are the hero of your own life's story, and by the time you reach the end of it—for it is, after all, a short ride—you will want to be as love-worn as the Velveteen Rabbit.

—Patrice Rancour
December, 2007
Columbus, Ohio, USA

1

Blythe Spirit in the Medical Intensive Care Unit

I no sooner turn on the pager, than it whines back at me.

Six forty-five a.m. and we have lift off, I mumble to myself. I switch my computer on in the storage closet that masquerades as my office, the space I share with two other clinical nurse specialists. As I dump my purse into the lower right-hand drawer, the computer screen comes alive with a list of messages to be replied to since yesterday. I choose instead to return the page, listening to the distress on the other end of the line.

"Can you come over to MICU right now? Mrs. Bueter just died and her husband is losing it over here."

As I slip on my lab coat, I make a note to myself that it is time to get a new one. I notice once again that it is frayed around the collar and cuffs. Every few months I seem to register this but still don't remember to do anything about it.

On the way to the intensive care unit, I pass by windows that I probably won't think to look through the rest of the day. The rain distorts them in streaming gray teardrops.

I consider the Bueters. How much they have gone through. All those weeks in the bone-marrow transplant unit, the massive infections that left her debilitated, the dire drug side effects that left her demoralized. And still she and her husband powered through. Denial is a wondrous thing, whether it comes from the patients or the medical staff.

I pass through a labyrinth of corridors, peering into rooms where I know nightmares are unfolding. What is it that Helen Keller noticed for us all? Was it that the world is full of suffering, and also the overcoming of it? I hope to God that this morning I can align myself with the last part of that equation. Some days, amidst all the suffering here, I have to wonder.

I push past the double doors into the medical intensive care unit and slide my frayed sleeves up to lather at the sink. In the flurry of the early morning shift change in the long MICU ward, I notice that one cubicle has its flowered bedside curtains completely drawn around it. No invasive procedure going on in there, I think. No intubation, no extensive dressing change, no catheterization. I know that on the other side of those curtains, two souls wait. One watching to make sure no harm comes to the other. The other is now Mr. Bueter.

"Mr. Bueter," I murmur softly as I slip through the curtains. "May I join you?"

He looks up at me, eyes glazed, and nods. Passively, he allows me to embrace him. His lax body is exhausted. Last night was the culmination of the three and a half months I have walked with both of them through this whole ordeal. And of course, it does not begin to address their previous two and a half years spent in diagnosis and treatments. All of which brings us to this time, this place.

We don't say much in the beginning. I look at him in profile. Although he is 52 years old, he looks 82. He is staring down at the body of his wife, to whom he had been married for 28 of those 52 years. As a result of their relationship, there are three others in this world, and one of them has two children.

As I sit with him, I try to imagine what this moment must be like for him. I say, "Robert, I am trying hard to imagine what this moment must be like for you. Help me understand what you are feeling."

He inhales a tremulous breath and silent tears course down his worn cheeks. Like the rain on the windows I passed on my way to the MICU, I think. He lets me take his hand. We sit that way for awhile, and I wonder if the description the nurse gave me about his "losing it" was really a description of her state of mind, her facing the start of another day in the MICU, a place where they are supposed to be saving lives.

After a bit, he wipes the tears from his face and pries one of those inadequate little tissues out of the hospital tissue box. During hospitalizations, when bodily fluids are predictably known to be more copious, more relentless, why are hospital tissues so notoriously stingy?

"She was a fighter," is all he says. He says it with admiration

I feel such a tender sadness when he says this. Truth, justice, and the American way. To be a fighter. Whatever the cost. Whether it makes sense to fight or not. A fighter to the end. Ours is a very macho culture, I think sadly.

Not so long ago, at a conference in New York, a World Health Organization official clucked his tongue at the audience, and shook his head. "You Americans. With your 'fighting' spirit, your 'war' on cancer, your 'armamentarium' of drugs. Do you not understand that most of the rest of the world understands that illness and pain are just a normal part of life?"

While this is true, what is also true is that due to the quintessential American refusal to smell bad, to suffer the slings and arrows of pain and illness, to our massive refusal to lay down and not go so gently into that good night, we now have tools like the polio vaccine, migraine headache medication, and organ replacement surgery. Of course, as these innovations come down the pike, they have often brought with them the kinds of ethical dilemmas that outstrip our technical abilities to cope with them. It is a mixed bag now, isn't it? The public always expecting that high tech will save them when it is many times that the high-tech solutions merely create the portal to the next nightmare that hadn't yet been anticipated.

I bring myself back to the present, to Robert Bueter. I notice that I am breathing rhythmically, a little habit I have become more conscious of in times of suffering. By matching the breathing of the one with whom I am sitting, and gradually and ever-so-gently lengthening the exhalations, we end up sitting in synchrony and breathing together. It is a way of bearing the deep ache of a broken heart, and doing it together.

Often, the only way into a heart is that it be broken first.

I turn my attention to Dorothy, Dorothy of the fighting spirit. Dorothy who fought because that was what was expected of her, from her family, from her doctors. She fought because no one she listened to offered her a different—

although no less honorable—option. Her body is filled with the fungus that overwhelmed her. And now that fungus is dying too. Kill the host, you kill yourselves, I think to myself. I can't help but think Dorothy and her greedy, fungal stowaways are a microcosm of what we are doing on a planetary scale. The world in a grain of sand.

I breathe myself back to the here and now, to Dorothy, knowing she is no longer in there. I believe with all my heart that Dorothy is most likely lingering around, and is kicking up her heels to be outside of this decaying vessel, her body, like a butterfly escaped from the confines of her cocoon. I think to myself, "You go, girl!" A small smile twitching the corners of my mouth as I picture her, mostly wishing she could let Robert know she is free at last. Free at last, free at last, thank God almighty, free at last!

And then, as if he is picking up my thoughts, Robert says, "You know, I think I can hear her whispering in my ear."

"Really, Robert? What is she telling you?"

"She says she is doing all right and not to worry about her."

"Do you believe her?"

"I believe her. It's just that I miss her so much already. It feels like someone has just opened my chest and removed my heart. I can't imagine my life without her." He drops his head into his hands.

But what is the old saying: Women grieve; men replace? I think—not unkindly—that Robert will most likely be remarried within the year.

Instead, I say, "While you are in the middle of this right now, it is hard to remember that Dorothy's illness was really just a small part of a much larger life. Right now, it seems like it was the totality of her life. But remember, Robert, it wasn't."

He dries his eyes and nods. "I know it."

"And so what was it that made you fall in love with Dorothy in the first place?"

His face gradually lightens with a wistful smile, despite the tears on his stubbled cheeks. "It was the first week of college, and I went to a pledge party at my roommate's fraternity. And as I walked in the door, there she was. I wasn't able to take my eyes off of her." I watch as his eyes fasten on some other time, some other place. They dart about as he retrieves shreds of his lived life, a waking, lucid dream.

"Love at first sight?"

"Well, for me, anyway" he replies, wiping the tears off his face, blowing his nose. "It took me the whole damned party to work up the nerve to go up to her and introduce myself." He looks down at the corpse of his wife and gently caresses what little hair she has back from her face. "You wouldn't be able to tell from looking at her now, but she was some kind of looker back then." I see him look at her, but know he is seeing the girl at the party instead.

I look at the body on the bed. It is bloated, cooling, mottled, the lips becoming dusky. Large bruises still track up and down her arms, her veins having blown long ago, despite the central line. I know the silent blood is already pooling by gravity into her back, her buttocks, the heels of her feet. I try to imagine the girl he is now seeing in his mind's eye. Instead, I catch a glimpse of a blithe spirit dancing rapturously in the cubicle above our heads.

"And so, is that how it began?"

He nods, time traveling to a point when there were no central lines, no low blood counts, no immunosuppressive drugs. His face youthens momentarily as he bridges back to a point on a timeline that has none of this devastation in it.

"Yeah," he smiles weakly at me. "And as they say, the rest is history."

"Robert, she was surely lucky to have you."

And he says with predictability, "No. I'm the lucky one." They all say that. Or nearly all of them.

It is always humbling to be in the company of such trust, such devotion, such love. It happens daily, but because it is so quiet, people do not appreciate how heroic it is. It doesn't show up in newspaper headlines. It will never be the lead story on the six o'clock news. But it is heroic nonetheless.

I meet his gaze and say levelly, "Robert, I see what you have done here. You were nothing short of remarkable with Dorothy."

He nods in acknowledgement, squeezing my hand.

"Thank you," he says gratefully. And I know he means it. It is no small thing to be caught in the act of doing something good.

My pager goes off again. I switch it to vibrate. He nods, acknowledging that my day is moving along as well as his, although now our paths must of necessity diverge. Each of us has our work cut out for us.

He suddenly turns to me and says, "How do you do this all day long, day after day?"

"Robert, of the two of us, yours is the harder job."

He shrugs and nods at the truth of this.

"Is there someone you would like me to call for you right now?"

"No. I just want to be able to sit here alone with her for awhile. Before all the business of having to bury her starts."

I nod, and we embrace, both of us knowing that this is most likely the last time we will see each other. I will try to get time off to go to Dorothy's funeral, but I know it is wise not to promise anything. It always depends on the workload, who calls in sick, and so on and so forth. I take one backward glance at the two of them, framed in the canopy of bed curtains pulled to protect the other patients from contemplating their own mortality. Who is the staff trying to kid? Everyone conscious knows what is happening behind those curtains.

2

THE MOST BEAUTIFUL GIRL IN THE WORLD

I go to the nurse's station, which is already humming and underway with the next shift's slate of crises, to return the page I had silenced.

"Hey, it's me," I say into the receiver. "What's up?"

"Yeah, it's about Marianne in 942. You promised her you would be here when they came by to take the dressing off her bilateral mastectomy. They're waiting on you."

"Be right over."

As I leave the intensive care unit behind me, I pass a lovely Somali woman swathed in her beautiful Muslim silks, her sneakers incongruously peeking up from under the exotic drapery. The bucket of hospital disinfectant she pushes ahead of her does nothing to diminish her elegance and dignity. We make silent eye contact as she slips by and nods imperceptibly, leaving a vaporous disinfectant trail in the air after her.

The hallway in front of the elevator bank is glutted with the morning traffic. Instead of waiting, I push through the stairwell door and decide that—for my own good— I should be using the stairs more often anyway. By the fourth floor, I am huffing and puffing. By the time I get to the landing on 9 South, I have broken a sweat.

As I approach Marianne's room, James, cradling the phone on his shoulder at the nurse's station, catches my eye.

"Here," he says, handing me a mirror while he packs a sheaf of papers into the pneumatic tube, "You're going to need this. Thanks for coming. I'll be in as soon as I get this stat order filled."

I nod.

"She's pretty ragged around the edges," he says. The rest of what he intended to say is interrupted by the voice coming to the phone on the other end of the line. He resumes his attention to the phone, asking for the piggy back IV solution that Margaret Eversole in room 922 needs.

I momentarily pause outside 942, praying that as I enter into the nightmare behind this door, I will somehow know what to say, how to direct my energies. I start the breathing as I push open the door.

The room is packed with people in white lab coats crowding around the bed. The corners of the room are still lost in the early morning darkness, but the harsh fluorescent overbed light, buzzing its low vibrational hum, is unforgiving as it carves out the figure in the bed in bright bold relief. A patient controlled analgesia pump, a device that automatically drips intravenous fluid into patients, is beeping in the room next door, equally merciless in its insistence.

"Wish someone would get to that damn pump already," Marianne grimaces as Charlene, the resident, pulls at the corner of the dressing across her chest. "Thanks for coming," she says to me. "I thought maybe you wouldn't get here in time."

I take her hand. "Wild horses…" I trail off and give her hand a squeeze. Her unruly blonde hair tells me she was doing a lot of tossing and turning in the night. Charlene continues to work at the dressing.

"How's the pain been?" I ask.

"Oh, not too bad," she minimizes. "Maybe a five or a six." Her pasty expression tells me a different story.

"We can do better than that," Charlene murmurs as she continues to work the paper tape gently around the dressing. Once the tape has been released, the medical students press forward, hovering over the operative site. No one is talking to Marianne or looking at her face, which is fairly drained of its strength, the mouth set resolutely, the eyes glassy. Charlene begins to lift the dressing when I realize I am holding my breath because everyone else, including Marianne, is holding theirs.

"Wait," Marianne says, a little too loudly. "Wait just a little bit, can you?"

Charlene looks into Marianne's face and nods, rising up a little bit, her latexed hands still on the dressing. Everyone in the room breathes a bit, including me.

I look into Marianne's eyes, eyes I have been staring into on and off for the past month as the 32-year-old single woman has worked through the shock and awe of a recurrence of her breast cancer from six years ago. Those eyes had been so resolute back then when she had heard for the first time that the recommendation was for a bilateral mastectomy. "They are not separating me from my girls," she had vowed at the time.

We seem to have time-traveled together in a split nanosecond as we both recognize what this moment means.

"You've come a long way, baby," I smile softly at her. "Well, are you ready?"

She nods at me. "I am." She looks back up at the resident, takes a deep breath, and says in a stronger voice, "You can go ahead now."

The resident gently lifts the dressings off and Marianne intently looks at the faces of all those medical students staring at her empty chest, watching their expressions with just as much concentration as I am watching hers.

A couple of them nod. "It looks great," one of them remarks. I wonder if it would look as great on his mother's chest, his sister's, his girlfriend's.

Charlene checks the integrity of the suture line and the two drains. "Marianne, everything looks the way it is supposed to here. Dr. Mack really did a nice job." She throws the old dressing into a nearby waste basket and starts to rip open a new dressing from a sterile package. "Did you want to take a peek before we dress it again?"

Marianne catches her eye. "Yeah, I do, but not with an audience. Do you mind giving me some privacy? Won't take me long."

Charlene smiles at her and places the dressing package back on the overbed table. "Honey, I've got a floor of patients to see. Take all the time you want." She removes her gloves and shoots them into the basket. "Come on boys and girls." She turns and threatens with mock gusto, "I'll be back."

They leave the room unceremoniously, closing the door behind them. We have been planning this moment since before the surgery. I take a scented candle out of her drawer and clear a space for it on the perpetually cluttered bedside table.

"I hope to God the sprinklers don't go off." I light the candle. The heady fragrance of jasmine begins to suffuse through the antiseptic gloom. Marianne flips on her CD and Pat Matheny's guitar licks light up the room. I turn on a softer incandescent lamp at the bedside, which means we no longer need the glare of the fluorescent light. As I turn it off, Marianne raises the head of her bed to about 30 degrees. I hold the mirror in one hand, waiting for her signal that she is ready to proceed.

"Before I look," she says looking me dead in the eye. "I want you to describe to me in detail what you see first. No whitewashing."

I meet her gaze evenly. "OK," I say as I scan her chest closely. "But let's work on the pain thing first. You want to bolus yourself before we do this?"

She nods as she reaches for the PCA button, and we hear the little ping as the morphine is released. Thank God for patient-controlled analgesia. In this entire mess, it is one of the few ways Marianne can control what is happening to her. Within moments, the muscles across her forehead visibly let go.

I continue. "It's like this. Each incision is about five inches long, running from each arm pit to your breastbone at about a ten-degree angle. The skin at the incision site is pink, of course, but not too bad. The suture line is pretty clean with nothing oozing from it to speak of. Each incision has its own drain, and the drains are doing their job pretty well with about a quarter of a cup of bloody drainage in each. Have you decided on names yet?" I ask the question as if she were naming her twins. In a way, she is.

"Yeah, I couldn't decide if I should name the drains Bert and Ernie, Hekyll and Jekyll, or Fred and Barnie."

"Well what have you settled on?"

"Lucy and Ethel," she says. "Remember, we're all girls here."

"So named," I say, and I knight each drain with a slight tap of my finger. "Anything else you want to know before you take a peek?"

She searches my face carefully.

"I don't think so," she says, so I hand her the mirror. She tries to bolus herself again, but we both know it is too soon.

"Well, here goes," she says, taking the mirror from me and holding it up to her mutilated chest. Her face registers nothing as her eyes search out what she sees in the mirror.

"Well, it's pretty much like you said," she murmurs.

"Remember, Marianne, you have a body, but you are more than just a body." I feel compelled to say this to her, thinking to buffer the shock.

"Actually, it looks just like I thought it would. I'm glad we spent all that time looking at mastectomy pictures before the surgery. And I'm really glad I'm not doing any reconstruction for awhile. I just don't think I could face all of that right now. And thanks for being honest with me. About how this looks." A tear slides down her left cheek. "I think I'd like to be alone right now for awhile if you don't mind."

"You sure?"

She nods. "I'm sure."

"I'll tell James to make sure he knocks before coming back and to make sure nobody else comes in. How much time do you need?"

"Oh, say about twenty minutes?"

"You got it. " I lean over and give her a careful squeeze. "Remember, it will not always feel like this," I tell her. Again, she nods. As I reach the door, I turn and say, "Oh, and make sure you blow out that candle before you let him back in here. Otherwise there will be three of us brought up before the fire marshal instead of just the two of us."

She looks back at me from the soft, scented light of her bed, and I think I have never seen anything quite so beautiful.

I bump into James as he walks out of the room next door, finally having put us all out of our misery by attending to the pump in question. I tell him about Marianne, and he nods.

"How's it going in there?" I point into the room he is leaving.

"Go on in and see for yourself," he grins.

"What's that smile for?" I ask suspiciously. "She was really a mess yesterday."

"Like I said, go in and see for yourself," and he saunters down the hallway, his corn-rowed plaits swinging smugly behind him.

3

THE MIDNIGHT VISITOR

I push open the door and whisper, "Mrs. Gomez, are you awake enough for a visit?"

"Come on in," she says.

She is sitting up in bed, sipping gingerly from a steaming Styrofoam cup of strong coffee. The aroma is fragrant. Gotta get me one of those, I think.

"Wow, you look like you are feeling a whole lot better than you were yesterday," I observe, approaching her bed. I can hardly believe the transformation. Yesterday, she was having a hard time coming to terms with learning that her tumor was not responding to the chemo. She had been so severely agitated she had been given a tranquilizer to try to calm her. This morning, I am with a different woman, one who has already carefully applied lipstick and who is, as they say in accepted hospital parlance, "in no acute distress."

"What's happened since I last saw you?" I ask, sincerely curious.

She smiles a knowing smile and focuses just above and to the right of me. I look around my shoulder, wondering if someone has just padded silently into the room, but there is no one there. Her gaze is persistent, and I try to step into it so we can resume eye contact. When I do so, her eyes flicker to the left of me. It is a bit unsettling.

"Well, yesterday, as you know, was a very hard day for me. When they told me they could not give me any more chemo or radiation, I lost it. I don't think I have ever felt so low in my life. And let me tell you, I've been low!" She sipped thoughtfully from the cup. "I just did not know if I could continue with all this suffering. And then last night, Jesus came to me, and laid his hand on my head, and told me he would take care of me, no matter what." Now she is finally looking directly right at me, "And ever since then, I have been just fine. Because I believe him." She looks back at the space above my upper shoulder and smiles knowingly.

Stepping back to resume eye contact, I say, "I'm really relieved that you've found some peace in all of this. I know you were in a lot of pain yesterday."

Suddenly, the obvious hits me and I realize what is happening here. I look at her pointedly.

"He's still here, isn't he? Jesus, I mean."

She nods, smiling into her coffee. I understand now that I have been stepping on another's toes, as I have been shifting position back and forth. I laugh at myself.

"Please forgive me," I grin at the space over my shoulder. She grins, too.

"Mrs. Gomez, I'm so very happy for you. " And truly I am, for when all hell is breaking loose around you, having faith such as this is nothing short of a miracle. And in her case, a real healing. "Do you want to talk about it?"

"No, I don't need anything right now," she says, quietly fingering the crucifix at her throat. "I am really very good. I am just very hungry today and want to eat."

"I can see that," I say, remembering that her appetite has been problematic the last week or so. Let's not mess with success.

I leave her waiting for her breakfast to arrive. Over the brim of her coffee cup, she continues to smile up at a face I am not privy to see. I chart what she has told me, and already can hear her doctors chalk it up to the morphine, a vacuous explanation at best, a regrettable lack of faith on their part at worst.

4

THE DIFFICULTY WITH LETTING GO

It is about then that I hear a disturbance down the hallway and start making my way toward the locus of the noise. As I approach the nursing station where the fracas is coming from, I see one of our attending physicians, stethoscope carelessly slung around his neck, standing in the hallway with an angry woman who is shouting into his face. He is listening to her calmly enough, but I sense he is reaching the end of his patience with her.

The woman is dressed rather plainly, in clothes that look as though they've seen better days. She appears to be in her early 60s, with mousy, graying hair, and a hard edge set to her face.

"I don't care if you think he's on death's door this very minute. I'm telling you I will sue you for every nickel you have if you do not pull him through this. You people charge enough for what you do here. *So do something!*" she shouts.

"I can see you are upset, Mrs. Bishop, but it doesn't change anything," said the resident. "Your husband does not want any further aggressive treatment here.

And while he is in his right mind, and he is my patient, I have to defer to him. It is his decision, not yours."

Other patients and family members come to the entrance of their rooms to see what all the commotion is about, but once they see what is happening, they disappear back behind closed doors. People have enough to deal with here without having to be party to the crises of others. This misery usually does not love company.

"So you think for as sick as he is, he's in his right mind? You're telling me he is actively dying, yet you think he can make up his own mind?" She is standing almost on tiptoe to be able to look him in the eye.

"Yes, Mrs. Bishop, that is exactly what I'm telling you. And if you don't keep your voice down, I'm going to have to ask you to leave the unit. You're beginning to upset the other patients here."

"Are you threatening me, Doctor?"

"Can we go down the hall to have this conversation privately?" he suggests.

She begins another explosive deluge of epithets. He begins to lose his patience with her and nods to a nurse behind the nurse's station.

"If you do not calm down, Mrs. Bishop, I will ask Stacy here to call security to escort you off the unit. Now I don't want to do that, but I can't have you upsetting everyone else here."

"Oh, *you* can't have? *You* can't have? Somebody ought to remind you that you work for *me*, doctor. And not the other way around."

At this, a younger man comes out of a nearby room and approaches her quietly but firmly.

"Mother, let's take a break now. You're getting yourself all worked up. Let's go out and get a cigarette." He reaches slowly for her arm, but she moves away from him.

"You're right, John, I do need a cigarette!" She turns to the attending. "You'd better not be here when I get back. I want another doctor for my husband. If you can't help him, maybe somebody else can."

As she stalks off the unit, her chagrined son in tow, the doc is left standing there, just shaking his head. I approach him.

"You handled that well, Richard."

"You're kidding, right?" he says.

"No, I'm not kidding. She was being quite difficult. What's the story?"

He walks me over to the nurse's station where we can have more privacy.

"Well, I really feel sorry for her poor husband. He is beginning multiple organ system failure and has been consistent about not wanting anything aggressive done for him. His kidneys are shot, his liver is shot, his heart and lungs are going. He wants to go home with hospice, but his wife there is in full-blown denial and is just not hearing him."

"Poor guy," I agree. "Anything I can do?"

"Yeah, if you want, go on in and support him. My guess is that this is the way she's been all her life and she's decompensating now. She seems to have poor coping skills. My guess is

21

that you won't make much in the way of in-roads with her in the short time he's got."

He gets up to write his notes. "Anything you can do to support the poor guy would be a good idea so he can get some peace and quiet. She's unreasonable, and I really think she's not rowing with all her oars in the water."

"I'll do what I can," I say, but add as an afterthought, "It's hard to remember that while she's screaming into your face, what you are probably dealing with is her grief reaction."

"That and a massive personality disorder," he smiles as he shakes his head. It's hard to have sympathy for a person who has just threatened to sue you for trying to take care of her dying husband.

I leave the station and knock on the patient's door. I hear a "come in," and I enter. An elderly man is lying on his side, his withered head cupped in his gnarled hands.

"I don't hear anything else going on out there. Is she gone?"

"Yes she went out with your son for a cigarette."

He shakes his head wearily. "Well, pull up a chair while we have some peace. My name is John Bishop."

I pull up a chair to the bedside and introduce myself. He pulls a sip from the straw in the cup of water at his bedside and wipes his mouth with the back of his hand.

"Your wife is a formidable woman, John."

"She's been that way her whole life. She's having a hard time accepting that I'm not going to recover from this illness.

It's making it hard for me to just let go. I'm worried about how my family will cope with her when I'm not there."

"Who all is in your family, John?"

"Well, there's Shirley, my wife—you just met her—and my two sons, John Jr. and Ted. And then there's my daughter, Sandy."

"Sounds like your wife gives you all a run for your money."

"Oh yeah," he says grimly. "She's a control freak. Always has been. Always will be. And this here situation is sending her right over the edge."

"So you think because she won't give you permission to let go, you're abandoning your family if you do?"

"That's exactly what it feels like," he says. "You know I'm mighty tired of just hanging on here. I keep hoping she's going to see the light, but I just don't see her being able to. She's always counted on me being the rock, you know. I don't think she believes she can handle things without me."

At that moment, Shirley comes flying back into the room. When she sees me, her eyes narrow suspiciously.

"Who are you and what are you doing here with my husband? I bet he's telling you what a witch he has for a wife now, isn't he?" She looks at him pointedly. "Forgot my damn cigarettes," she mutters as she grabs them from a coat pocket thrown over a chair. "You know, I just might go down there and throw myself in front of a damn truck!" And with that, she stomps out of the room.

He looks at me helplessly. "You see what I'm working with here?"

"Is she likely to follow through with that threat?"

"Naw, it's mostly for show."

"Well, John, the way I see it, your wife's not as helpless as she makes you all believe she is."

"Well, Shirley's always been a little on the head-strong side."

"So what do your sons and daughter say about all this?"

"They tell me to do what I need to do. That they're all right."

"Well, do you believe them?"

"Oh, I guess I do. They're good kids. It's just that I feel a little guilty leaving them here to deal with Shirley. I've kind of buffered them from her all their lives."

"Well, it's not like they're kids anymore," I observe. "And, I don't know how much you've really been able to buffer them. I saw your son out there with his mother and he seemed to handle himself pretty well."

"Well, I guess that's true enough," he says thoughtfully.

"You know, John, you give a lot of your power away to Shirley, don't you?"

"What do you mean?"

"I mean, she's not here now. You've got your kids' permission to let go. You've got permission from all of us here to let go. And yet you don't let yourself. The only permission you really need is the permission you're denying yourself."

"You think it's easy as all that?"

"I didn't say it was easy. But maybe it's just that simple."

"I never much looked at it that way."

I can't suppress the smile that hovers at my lips.

"What's so funny?"

"I think you're afraid she's going to be so mad at you for having the nerve to leave her that she's going to come after you and make your life just as miserable in the hereafter."

With that, he grins back at me. "You know, young lady, I do believe you're right." And he takes another little sip from his straw.

I rise from the chair and shake his hand. "Well, John, it has been a pleasure to have met you. I just want you to know that I have every confidence in you that when you are truly ready, you will take the next right step."

"Well, thank you for your time here today. I won't forget it."

I leave the room. All seems quiet in the hallway for now, although I am pretty sure there will be more fireworks once someone has finished her cigarette. I wonder if John's wife will let me in, will let me help her with this. I'd also like to think that John will give himself the permission he needs and not be here tomorrow when it will start all over again. I'll try to remember to check the census when I get in. I can't help but wish him bon voyage.

5

DYING FOR LOVE

I glance at my watch, realizing that my outpatient appointment with the Jablonski's is rapidly approaching, and I need to find space to meet with them since my office is neither big enough nor private enough. In a hospital, space is a four-letter word. Luckily, I locate an empty office just off the lobby right as I get the call they have arrived.

I begin to shift from Bishop to Jablonski mode as I descend the stairwell. Interesting couple, the Jablonski's. When Karen had been diagnosed with her stage three cancer, it seemed to suit her just fine. She had been lost in a loveless relationship with husband Mike for the past 19 years. She was pretty well worn out from it. Hence, the cancer, I had wondered? A few people will look for a more socially acceptable way out of a bad relationship, preferring illness to divorce, or worse.

Not that Mike had been overtly abusive—just basically loveless, indifferent, and emotionally unavailable until Karen was diagnosed. At which time he apparently transformed into a remarkably caring husband who pulled out all the stops for her. It became evident that he understood how much she meant to him about the time he thought he was going to lose her. He became attentive, caring, and—dare I use the word?—*doting*. Under his care, she blossomed, despite the rigors of intensive treatment. She finally received what she had been missing for 19 years: a loving relationship.

The chemo treatments continued, until at a certain point about six months ago, Karen's physicians had told her that they had no further curative treatment available for her, that it was time to get her affairs in order, as the saying goes. They did have one last clinical trial they could enroll her in, but they didn't hold out much hope it would do much for her. Still, for her, it represented the last resort. At this point, Karen had decided she didn't want to die after all. She finally had her husband back. She decided to go for it. And, by God, she did. And, under Mike's care, don't you know that her last two scans proclaimed of her, "no evidence of disease."

It was an amazingly unexpected outcome—something that her doctors chalked up to "spontaneous remission," as they scratched their heads and put her on a surveillance program. It might have been "spontaneous," but I didn't see anything mysterious about it. It hadn't been the chemo that was making the difference for Karen. It had been Mike. That had been about four months ago, and last week, she had called for a tune-up appointment with me. I am really looking forward to this appointment. In this line of work, inhaling all the really good news one can get helps to get through the difficult days.

I spot the Jablonski's in the lobby and wave for them to follow me down the corridor where the consultation room is waiting for us. I notice that Karen is looking rather glum, but decide to dismiss it from my awareness. I am needing a party here. Good news.

As I close the door behind us, and we each take our seats, I notice that the couple decidedly choose not to sit together on the only couch in the sparsely-appointed consultation room. Uh-oh, I think, as I plow ahead with, "How are things going?"

Karen is looking down into her empty hands, her dishwater blond hair draping her face so that I cannot make out her expression. Mike is carefully examining the blank wall above my head. I wait out the silence. Karen starts weeping, keeping her head low, hiding behind her hair. Mike looks at her in a detached manner, reminding me of how they had initially presented the day I first met them. I continue to wait them out.

Karen is mumbling something unintelligible. I look pointedly at Mike who is visibly trying to avoid eye contact.

"He's doing it again," she murmurs finally.

"What's that?" I ask, although it doesn't take a rocket scientist to see what is happening here.

"She's trying to tell you—I'm back," he says in a sing-song sarcastic voice.

"Go on," I prompt.

He is cool, detached, not to be moved, and in his own passive-aggressive way, exasperating.

He shakes his head and clams up. I am still waiting them out.

Karen wipes her face, takes a deep breath, and finally looks up at me. She looks like she did when we first met months ago—older than her chronological age.

"He is treating me the way he did before," she reports sadly. "Ever since the doctor told me that I am cancer-free, we are back to the way we were before. I can't believe it. I just cannot believe it."

I look at Mike's face and have to agree with his wife. Now that she is safe and sound, he seems to have retreated back to the old status quo before her diagnosis. I thought this man had finally received his wake-up call and had in fact "gotten it." But, I guess that is not what is happening here after all.

I can't help but feel exasperated with Mike. Neither one of them is looking at me, so the three of us sit in silence.

"Really, I don't know what she wants from me anymore," Mike whines. "She is back like she was before. So what does she want from me anyway?"

"Not this!" she mutters.

"You know," I say, "I'm having a flashback right now to about a year ago, to a different patient who told me that she would prefer to be in the hospital with her cancer diagnosis than to be at home with her alcoholic husband. You are both reminding me of someone else who confided in me last week that she believed it wasn't her cancer killing her, but her marriage. And that as soon as she could get her cancer addressed, she was getting out of a very bad relationship. Is this ringing any bells for the two of you?"

They look at their opposing walls. I feel like I am the referee in a ring. I don't want to be a referee, and I surely do not want to be in this ring.

"Look, the way I see it is that you have three choices," I continue. "You can go on doing this the way you did it before. You can do something different and stay together. You can split up. So what's it going to be?" I seem to have run out of patience.

"This isn't very helpful," Mike says to me.

"What do you think would help?" I ask.

"Not this."

I consider my next words carefully. "Mike, don't you see how powerfully healing your love for Karen is?"

I catch his eye briefly before he looks up again to the spot over my head. Personally I am hoping it is the halo I am earning that he is staring at.

"You know," I continue, "the docs believe that it was the chemo that cured Karen. Even though they told you initially that they didn't believe it would have much of an effect. But you know, I don't believe for a minute that it was the chemo. Do you?"

He squirms around a bit in the too-small chair. "What do you want me to say?" he asks, still guarded, although his voice has just dropped an octave. I pursue it.

"What is it that *you* want to say, Mike?"

He doesn't say anything for a long time, but when he looks at me, his eyes are just the slightest bit glassy.

"I guess I'm protecting myself."

"From...?"

"From having to go through all of this all over again," he says this with no expression, but his voice breaks.

"The 'this' being?" I ask him.

He breaks. "All of this," he says, gesturing widely with his arms. "This damn place. The whole thing. Having to face— you know," he gestures vaguely in Karen's direction.

She is looking at him steadily now.

"No, I don't know," she says evenly. "Having to face what exactly?"

"The possibility that I could lose you—still, yet, again, whatever," he responds, not able to meet her gaze, waving his hand back and forth dismissively.

"Why couldn't you just tell me this, Michael? Why couldn't we just talk about it?"

"Too painful," he says, rubbing the center of his chest.

I notice this gesture and have a hunch about it. "Mike, what's going on in your chest right now?"

"It's a pressure. Heavy pressure. I just can't shake it."

"Is it your heart?" Karen asks, alarm in her voice. I know she is thinking heart attack, angina.

"Naw, nothing like that," he says still rubbing the center of his chest. "More like an ache."

"Actually, Karen, it is his heart. How long has that been going on?"

"Oh, ever since this whole damn thing with Karen started. I thought it would have gone away by now."

"Mike, could you just humor me right now?" I ask. "I'd like you to just gently press into the sore spot in your chest with your thumb. Yeah, you can go ahead and close your eyes. I'd like you to just breathe deeply into and out of that place you're probing with your thumb. Just take a nice deep breath. That is the initial signal breath. A signal to your body that we are moving into a special time and place set aside just for you. All other breaths will be breathed normally, peacefully, rhythmically."*

He begins to settle down, and I notice Karen is engrossed in the emerging scenario.

I continue. "You'll be hearing sounds from inside the room and sounds from outside the room. Nothing to change. Nothing to judge. Just allow your attention to move from one sound to the next. Breathing in and out, in and out. You'll be having thoughts about what has happened, what is happening now, what is going to happen. Nothing to change. Nothing to judge. Just detach from your thoughts and watch them as if they were a movie up on a movie screen. Because right now all you have to do is breathe."

The mood in the room shifts from one of hostile agitation to that of sincere absorption. It even smells differently. I wonder if that subtlety has to do with pheromones that have suddenly transitioned from fear to surrender. He was right there with all this just below the surface. So very little guardedness to plow through. I am surprised, yet grateful, that he is allowing this. His breath is slower, as is Karen's, as is my own. She is watching, clearly fascinated by Mike's willingness to permit himself to be so vulnerable. Timing is everything.

"As you continue to breathe, allow your conscious awareness to move to your heart space. This is the space in your

*This guided imagery approach is based on the work of Stephen Levine.

chest, where your heart resides. And as you move there with your awareness, continue to probe that space gently with your thumb, noticing any resistances or holdings or armoring of your heart. Noticing without judgment, without needing for anything to be different from the way it is. Breathing rhythmically, naturally, and peacefully."

Mike is exploring his chest with his thumb, searching ever so subtly the area just to the left of his breastbone. He is surprisingly focused for someone who presented with so much initial resistance.

"As you continue to breathe, allow your awareness to come to the place in your heart where the ache lives. Notice how all the tissues of your heart are attached to the ache, and begin slowly but surely to soften the connection between the heart and its ache. Softening all the tissues that keep the ache attached to it. As you breathe, soften, soften, soften. Melting the connection between the ache and the heart, until finally, and surely, the ache is floating free in the space you have just created for it. Nothing to change, nothing to judge, just allowing the ache to float free in the space in your heart."

Mike's face is much softer now. The breathing has steadied him and allowed him to explore his experience without fear. He has become his own scientific investigator.

"Now go to the place in your heart where your compassion for other people in trouble lives. You know where that is and where to go to find it. Breathe into that place now and notice that as you do so, your heart space becomes more expansive, more spacious, more caring. So expansive, that there is plenty of space there to put yourself in your own heart. And you do that right now."

33

As I say these words, silent tears course down his cheeks. Karen's, too, as she watches from the corner of the room. We sit there quietly like this for some time.

Then I say, "And now, using your breath as a conduit, breathe in the warmth of your heart space and exhale it into the space in your heart where the ache is floating free. Breathing in warmth, breathing out compassion. Breathing in love. Breathing out tenderness. Breathing in forgiveness and having a little mercy on yourself. Allow the ache to float free, bathed in the warmth of your forgiveness and compassion. Nothing to change. Nothing to judge."

Mike's breathing is like the ebb and flow of a deep tidal current, seeming to take him deeper and deeper. Being with him like this is a meditation for myself. And I realize that doing this on behalf of others is always like doing it for myself. The three of us breathing in unison, almost like the syncopation of silvery fish swimming in a school, turning in unison together as one organism. When it feels like we have been where we are for sufficient time—don't ask me how I know this—I continue.

"And now, very gently, very softly, begin to bring your conscious awareness back to this space, back to this time, taking with you as much as you can from this experience. Know that you can return to this experience any time you wish just by taking that initial signal breath. Know that you have the power to do so any time you wish and that you take that power with you everywhere you go. When you are ready, you can stretch and open your eyes."

It takes him awhile to open his eyes. When he finally does so, he lets his hand drop into his lap. He looks at both of us placidly, with a little surprise. He then gets up and sits next to Karen and puts his arms around her. The two of them sit like that softly weeping together for some time. I begin to wonder if I just should leave, as if my presence is unduly intrusive here in this intimacy. Just as I am thinking this, Mike gently peels himself from Karen's embrace, and turns to me while he takes her hand.

"Thank you for that," is all he says.

"You are very welcome," I say.

I turn toward Karen now. "At the risk of spoiling the moment, there is something I keep thinking that won't go away so it must mean that I am supposed to share it with you."

"What's that?"

"Karen, do you not see that you really do not have to die for Mike's love? That there are ways of finding peace other than dying?"

She looks down into her lap, and new tears flow. She nods, but there are no more words needed here. And now I do know that I am overstaying my welcome. I rise to leave, and motion for them to stay.

"I think the two of you need some time alone," I say. "Stay here as long as you want."

They both nod, and I nod back at them as I close the door behind me.

6

THE PARABLE OF THE OAK TREES

The appointment with the Jablonski's has drained me. I decide to go for that cup of coffee before something else happens. I also decide I owe myself an elevator ride down to the cafeteria. Miraculously, the elevator door opens just as I arrive. And who is grinning just behind the elevator doors but Nathan. Nathan Mintz. He welcomes me in the elevator with a hug.

"What are you doing back here?" I ask. "Can't stay away from us, can you? What are you, a glutton for punishment?"

He smiles softly, sweetly even. Nathan was Don Chaykin's son-in-law. And what a son-in-law! I never saw two men unrelated by blood closer than those two. Don died last week, and I did not expect to see Nathan back in the hospital.

"No, actually, I had to come back and pick up some things from the business office. And Edna had left a pair of reading glasses that the nurses on 7 were keeping for us. Thought I'd just swing by to pick them all up at the same time."

"How are Edna and Shelia doing through all this?"

The elevator stops and lets on a silent group of people who look exhausted. None of them says anything, just looking at the floor or looking up at the flashing crimson numbers with that glazed-over elevator stare. Someone's clothes are saturated with the acrid smell of cigarette smoke, and it is oppressive in the confining space. Nathan becomes reluctant to talk further now that our privacy has been breached, but I can see he would like to. The door opens to the front lobby; the people file silently out the door, their story trailing after them like the bitter tobacco smoke odor wafting behind them.

Nathan looks at me, somewhat tentatively. "Say, are you in a hurry to get somewhere?" he asks.

"Just to be with you," I reply.

"Can we go somewhere where we can talk?"

"Sure," I smile and the two of us approach Marvelle who sits at the reception desk with the phone crooked to her shoulder. She nods back without missing a beat, her eyes on her computer screen, giving hand directions to someone who is lost at the desk. When people who have never been here arrive, Marvelle is the first impression they have of us. She is our best foot put forward. Marvelle knows all. When the CEO wants to know what is going on in the hospital, he ambles down to the front lobby and chats with Marvelle.

Getting her attention, I make a silent turning gesture with my hand, and she riffles through a desk drawer to find the key to a private little room off the lobby where surgeons sometimes go to inform families of the "open and close" cases—the cases the medical students irreverently refer to as "peek and shriek." On more than one occasion, Marvelle has paged me with a "Can you come down here? Dr. so-and-so had to give some bad news to a family and they are having a bad time of it."

A lot of people lose a lot in this building.

Today, Nathan and I find sanctuary in the small room and shut off the busyness of the lobby behind us as the door closes. His dress is always casual but highly manicured. Even his jeans have creases in them. He has been very good to this family he married into. Because, as he likes to note, they have always been very good to him.

"I'm really glad I ran into you," he says. "Amazing things have happened since we last talked." Such an open face. He removes his glasses and rubs the lenses absently with a tissue before he puts them back on.

"I'm all ears," I encourage him.

"Did Edna tell you what happened with Don the weekend he died? And since then?"

"Actually, no. I don't think I've spoken to anyone in the family since Don died."

"I thought I hadn't seen you in awhile," he nodded. "Well, you know that Saturday night, he was up most of the night. Kept waking up Edna, saying, 'Why can't you turn out that light?' And Edna kept telling him there was no light, that it was the middle of the night and he should go back to sleep. But he kept covering his head with his arms and complaining about how bright the light was.

"The next morning, he is wide awake, and spunky. I mean like the Energizer Bunny or something. He tells Edna to call everybody in, that he needs to talk to everybody. So Edna does. Calls everybody in. And I think there must have been close to 35 people go through that room that whole day. Then around 5:00 p.m. we can see he is getting pretty exhausted. He agrees he can't visit much with folks anymore. When everybody leaves, he suddenly gets very tired. So he turns to me right before he settles down in bed and starts talking to me, saying strange stuff, really strange stuff. Telling me, 'be sure not to miss it, Nathan. It's between the third and fourth trees.'

"And I say back to him, 'Don, what are you talking about? What's between the third and fourth trees?' But he's already falling back into the pillows and muttering to himself about the trees. Pretty soon, he's asleep. And then of course, you know, several hours later, he's gone."

As I am watching him, Nathan's face is intense. He is powerfully focused, passionately engaged in the telling of his story. What is that old Alcoholics Anonymous maxim? *In the hearing is the learning, but in the telling is the healing*? He goes on.

"So, Edna, Sheila, and I are out the next day at the cemetery, making sure everything is okay with the plot. Don had wanted a shady double plot. You know how he loved his trees. So the cemetery representative says to us, 'Gee, it's too bad you folks didn't arrange this earlier. We just opened a new section in an area we call the grove. Your husband probably would have liked it, nice and shady as it is. The only plots we have open now up there are all out in the open.'

"And that's when the phone suddenly rings, and he says he's sorry he has to take it because he's been waiting on a call

all morning. He gets off the phone and says to us that we're in luck, that something has just opened up. Would we like to take a look at it? We say, sure, so he takes us in his car to an older section of the cemetery and tells us on the way that the couple who have been holding onto this particular plot decided to let it go since they have moved to be closer to where their children are living and have decided to stay out there to make it easier on everyone.

"Anyway, the long and the short of it is that as we drive around a curve in the road, we come along a line of big old oak trees. Beautiful, big old trees. And he slows down the car and points to the plot. And don't you know where it is?"

"Between the third and fourth trees?" I ask as if on cue.

He nods his head with a wondrous grin on his face.

"Well, gee, now, Nathan, you've got the hairs on the back of my neck standing straight up."

"Can you believe that story?" he asks with wonder.

"Without a doubt," I answer. "It sounds just like Don—taking care of business right up until the end."

"That's what I told Edna and Sheila, too."

He looks a little wistful and takes a deep breath. "You know he was like a father to me."

"Because you were like a son to him."

He nods in agreement. The wondrous thing about this work is that it allows me entrée into peoples' lives at their most intimate moments. I can walk into a room and because there are a series of little letters behind my name, people let me touch them. And the wondrous thing is that they touch me, too. In all sorts of ways.

There suddenly seems to be a detonation of noise outside the room. Sounds of people running, the overhead public address system muffled from outside the room, equipment clattering down the tiled corridor, its reverberation punctuated by a staccato rhythm. The moment is over. Nathan stirs, and we both stand up.

"I am so glad I ran into you," he says, and we embrace warmly.

"So am I," I tell him. "Give my best to Shelia and Edna, won't you?"

He nods and we head for the door. As we open it, the bustle of the lobby explodes into what had been our little world, and that moment is gone.

"See ya," he says as he turns to go.

"Yeah, see ya," I smile back to him, knowing once again that it is unlikely that I shall ever see him again—at least not in the way most people believe.

7

THE CODE IN THE LOBBY RESTROOM

Before I can even think my next thought, Marcey, the nurse manager for the clinic off the lobby, hooks my arm into hers and drags me over to the men's restroom.

"Boy, am I glad to see you," she says. "Leo McElroy just finished with his clinic appointment with Dr. Royce. He went into the restroom and the next guy in there finds him collapsed on the floor. They've just called a code, and the code team has just arrived. Can you take his wife over to exam room #2 and sit with her while they work on him?"

She does not wait for me to answer, but turns abruptly to an elderly woman who has shell-shock written all over her. Mrs. McElroy is a vision of gray. Gray raincoat, gray hat, gray face.

"Mrs. McElroy, this is Patrice, one of our clinical nurse specialists. While the code team is in with your husband, she will wait with you. Just go on down the hall with her, and we will get back in touch with you as soon as we can."

And with that, she turns down the hallway and is gone. There is some shouting in the bathroom as the door opens, and we see way too many people in a crowded space working on the floor around Mr. McElroy, who is not visible. Marcey has posted Linda, one of her patient care assistants, outside the restroom so that no one else can go in.

I take Mrs. McElroy by the arm, and she lets me direct her into the exam room. It is brazenly sterile, the light over the sink piercing, the air frigid. We both sit down on the hard chairs.

"Are things happening so fast you can't catch up with them?" I ask, a real gift for stating the obvious, I think.

She is in a state of wide-eyed wonder. "He was just fine. We were in with the doctor. And then he had to go to the restroom. I was just waiting outside the door. But he didn't come back out. I was waiting such a long time that I finally asked that nice young man to go in to see if he was all right. And then he came running back out, yelling for help."

"What did the doctor say during your visit?" I ask, thinking that if I keep her engaged, it will help with the mounting anxiety as the shock starts ebbing a bit.

"Well we both knew that Leo's cancer was terminal, but he checked out okay today. We were back in just for a change in his pain medicine, and to review his last scans. Nothing earth shattering. I can't believe this is happening. We were just in with the doctor. . ." Her voice trails off in disbelief.

"So you both understood that Leo's time was short?" I ask.

"Oh, yes. He had everything put in order. Didn't want to trouble me with any arrangements."

"Did he have a living will and durable power of attorney?" I inquire.

"Oh, yes, Leo was big on that. Said that he didn't want to prolong anything. That when his time came, that was it. He just wanted to be let go."

"Like right now?" I ask, feeling anxious about what is happening in the men's restroom at this very moment. In the fragmented world of modern health care, no one on a code team has ever set eyes on the person whose chest they are compressing, let alone understand what their end-of-life care preferences might be.

She looks at me, her eyes getting even bigger. "Why, yes, I guess right now. My God! But I'm not ready for this!"

"No one is ever ready, Mrs. McElroy. But tell me, if your husband were sitting here with us right now, what would he say he would want?" I look at her resolutely.

She looks back and I see she has made her decision. "He would say he would not want to be brought back," she says, just as determinedly.

"You're sure, Mrs. McElroy?"

"I'm sure," she says.

"I need to tell them right away. I'll be right back, okay?"

She nods. I run out of the room and plunge past Linda, slamming open the door, almost hitting the person standing behind it. "He has a living will," I yell into the pandemonium. "His wife says no resuscitation!"

This takes a few seconds to register. And then the resident in charge of the code comes up for air. "He doesn't want to be coded?"

"Yes, I've been speaking with his wife. Come verify if you need to."

He jumps over the gaggle of people on the floor and dashes with me back to the exam room. He listens as the dazed woman repeats what she has just told me.

"You're sure about this?" he asks.

By now, she is resolute. "Without a doubt," she responds.

He nods at me and rushes out the door. We hear him calling ahead of himself, "Call it. Stop the code. Call it!"

And suddenly, all the commotion comes to a stark halt. A few moments pass, and Marcey sticks her head in the door.

"Mrs. McElroy, we are bringing your husband's body to the exam room next door. I'll come back and get you when we are ready for you to be with him."

Mrs. McElroy looks up at her with disbelieving eyes. Was it only 20 minutes ago that they had left the doctor's office with a prescription in hand and an appointment card in the other? She is living in a temporal limbo. From now on, her life will be remembered from before this time and from after this time. I am very aware of the sanctity of this moment for her. This is what it means to be the witness at the crossroads of other people's lives.

Marcey's head disappears as she lets the door close gently behind her. Mrs. McElroy looks at me uncomprehendingly.

"This can't be really happening," is all she can say.

"This must be feeling surreal to you."

Her eyes search mine. "I wish I could wake up."

For the second time this morning I ask, "Is there someone you would like for me to call for you?"

She shakes her head slowly. "I just want to be alone with him right now, that's all. I have been preparing for this for some time, but I didn't see it happening like this. I thought it would be slower. I thought I would have more time. I thought . . ." Her words trail off.

We sit there together bound in the solemnity of her tragedy. She is so crushed, she cannot yet cry, but there will be plenty of time for tears soon enough. And I realize, again, how vulnerable we all are. Each of us. How fragile life is and that it can turn on a pin in a flash. Which is also what makes each moment so precious. After all, what is life, but just such moments, strung one after another, like dew on a spider's web, each glistening with its own particular light. Until by the very end, one can begin to see the pattern of the web as a whole. All the intersections, the interconnectedness of it all. Working here is like being in Life School, I think. And all these people have been brought into my life to be my teachers. Funny how they think I am here to help them.

And then the door opens, and Marcey is standing in its doorway. "Mrs. McElroy, we have your husband in the room next door. Are you ready?"

She stands up, more firmly than I expected, holding her purse tightly in both hands at her waist, and we follow Marcey into the next room. Mr. McElroy has been respectfully re-dressed and is lying on top of the exam table with a sheet up to his chest. I turn off the harsh overhead light and turn on the softer light above the sink. I turn to Mrs. McElroy who has eyes only for her husband.

"You girls can go on now," she says. "I need to talk to my husband."

Marcey and I look at her and back to each other.

"I'll be right outside, Mrs. McElroy, if you need anything," she says.

Mrs. McElroy does not say anything in acknowledgement, but waits for us to leave. I see her standing over the body of her husband, her fingers reaching for his face as the door closes behind us.

"You go on," Marcey says to me. "I've got this now."

"Are you sure?"

"I'm sure," she says, "but thank God you came out of that room when you did!"

I smile slightly in acknowledgment, and walk slowly back down the hallway, trying to remember where I was going when this whole thing started. When someone passes by me with a fragrant, steaming cup of coffee, I change direction and head down to the cafeteria, remembering I have a rendezvous with a similar cup.

8

Lessons in Powerlessness

In the elevator, there is an Indian couple. He's dressed in a western-style suit, very formal, and she is in a beautiful gold and rose sari. He is speaking in a heavily-accented voice, "No, no, no. We cannot do the procedure on that day. I tell you it is not a propitious day."

The woman turns to him and says quietly, "But, Binoy, the doctor says that she doesn't have the surgery room on the day you want. It's just not their way here."

"I am telling you, Mehdu, she will have to change the date or we cannot go through with it here. It is simply not a propitious day."

The elevator doors open and close behind me as I leave them to their wrangling. I truly hope the surgeon, whoever she is, is culturally competent and flexible enough to ask the OR to alter the surgery schedule on behalf of the patient in question.

I am standing in line when Joyce passes by me. You can't miss Joyce. She's almost ready to deliver her baby, and her bulbous belly parts the waves of people ahead of her long before the rest of her arrives. She stops suddenly.

"You hear what's happening upstairs?" she asks.

"Nope, haven't heard a thing."

"Marilyn's son is over in the SICU. Just brought him up there from the emergency room. Bad car accident. He was the passenger with another kid driving. Just got their driver's licenses."

I am out of line in an instant and heading to the elevator bank. None of them is anywhere close to this floor so I find myself once again bounding up the stairwell. When does all this running up and down the steps pay off in being more fit, I wonder. As I reach for the door handle and pull it wide open, I am anxious.

Marilyn is one of our top nurses on the step-down unit, one of those nurses who I would want taking care of me should I ever need it. Like other master nurses, Marilyn's clinical instincts are so sharp she cannot really tell you how she knows what she knows. She just does. And she is almost always right. The attending physicians never question her judgment. Her actions have saved them too many times.

I see activity in and out of the report room as I enter the surgical intensive care unit. When the door opens again, I see Marilyn sitting in the corner, talking quietly to someone in a suit whose back is to me. I walk into the room and sit across from her, catching her eye. She nods at me but does not stop answering the questions being posed by the representative from the local organ donor organization.

I watch the scene unfold as if I am an actress in some absurdist drama. None of this feels real to me. And if it doesn't feel real to me, how can Marilyn still be functioning inside this crazy play? Marilyn's son is the same age as my son. My identification with Marilyn is complete, and I am no longer in full control of myself. While I have called the organ donor program people for consultations with families of potential donors, I have never sat in on one of their interviews before. The sheer number of questions is mind-numbing.

"Has your son been outside the country in the last six months? To your knowledge, has your son ever taken injectable street drugs? To your knowledge, has your son had sexual relations with multiple partners?"

It goes on and on, and there's Marilyn facing the interviewer answering the deluge of questions as if it were reasonable to be doing so while her son is lying brain-dead in the room next door. The interviewer murmurs something apologetically and bends down to retrieve yet another form from his brief case. Marilyn looks over at me.

"Can you believe I am sitting here like this? Can you believe Joel is in the next room?" Her eyes are glassy, as are mine. I think I will explode with tears and fears about just how fragile we all are. That there is no good reason for this to have happened, and so on and so forth, while all along I know there is. I just don't happen to understand it.

I sit through the rest of the interview with her, and then it is time to get up and go to where Joel is. The curtains are closed, and there are a few family members who have already started to arrive, waiting for Marilyn to be the first to enter. She takes a deep breath, and I think, here again, a life will be remembered from before this moment and from after this moment.

I am anxious about how Joel's body will look. How bad the injuries will be. But as the drapes are pulled aside and we enter the cubicle, I think magically—like a child—"Why doesn't he just wake up?" Lying there on the SICU bed is the body of a beautiful 16-year-old boy. He is in that in-between place in adolescence when you can still make out what he looked like as a child, but you can already imagine him as the young man he is turning into, the angularity of maturation hardening the soft contours of his face. He looks perfect. He is without blemish. And he is brain-dead.

Marilyn is at once at the head of the bed cradling him in the anguished embrace of a Pietà sculpture. My identification is so complete that it is just too painful for me to stay. And as the tears come before I can hold on to them, I am out of that room, running away. I run into an empty corridor that has been closed for remodeling. And I cry and cry and cry. I cry for Marilyn. I cry for Joel. I cry for everyone. But most of all I cry for myself. Because my own son is 16, and he has just gotten his driver's license. And suddenly I am afraid of the world, and I feel powerless and know there is no way I was ever in control anyway. This is just another teaching sent to help jettison the illusion that I have any control whatsoever. I cry until I am exhausted. I know I should go back into that room, but I just can't face it right now. The caregiver guilt floods in: "Come on, stretch a little. Rise above it." But the fear pokes its fist into my chest and is squeezing my heart so hard, I can hardly breathe. And I think, thank God that we do not have to be all things to all people. And I judiciously— or cowardly—give myself permission not to go back. I am not so narcissistic as to think that in the midst of all her pain that Marilyn will miss me. Thank God there are other people in there with her now. I feel like a bucket that has just been emptied out.

Just as I am getting myself together and deciding that I can't hide out in this dank corridor forever, the pager goes off. I sigh deeply and understand that the universe is calling me back from my pity party to once again return to the world.

9

And Now It's Time for You to Stop Taking Yourself So Seriously

"It's me," I say, feeling like a wrung-out dish rag. I am hoping to God I'm in shape enough to do whatever I am about to be asked.

"I think you better come down here," Jackie says. "We've got a patient, and we can't figure out what his problem is."

"What do you mean?"

"Well, it'd just be easier if you were to get down here and see for yourself. He's in 1056."

"I'm on my way." I'm already curious and preparing myself for what is next on tap. As I make my way down the main hallway, I pass Diane who stops me.

"Do you have time to talk?" she asks. She's a young nurse with a ponytail; she's been here less than six months. Her lips are drawn in a taut line, and she looks tired, a little tightly wound, especially for someone so new. We try to keep an eye on the new ones because the nature of the work is so stressful here where we deliver bad news, not babies.

"Will you be around in the next hour or so? I'm on my way to a quick consult on the other station?"

"Sure," she says, looking away timidly.

"I promise, I'll come find you as soon as I'm finished," I reassure her.

She nods and stands in the hallway a bit forlornly. Wishing I didn't have to run away from her, I turn and ask, "Is this an emergency, Diane?"

The ponytail bounces from side to side as she shakes her head "no." Its perkiness stands in stark contrast to the rest of her.

"I'll be back as soon as I can."

I turn the corner and see a small group of nurses congregating at the station, Jackie among them. They are deep in conversation but stop as I approach.

"What's up?" I ask, sidling up to the group. "Can't imagine that you need me when you have such great minds at work here."

They look at me in earnest as Paul leans forward toward me and whispers, "It's Mr. Washington in 56. We can't figure out what's wrong with him. Yesterday he was fine, and today he is acting peculiar."

"Well, what's changed since yesterday?"

"He's started his chemo," Eunice with the gold front tooth explains. Eunice is a permanent fixture here. She's a woman with a lot of street smarts that the better educated among us lack.

"Well, maybe he's got a little delirium from the chemo—fluid and electrolyte imbalance already? Potassium maybe?

Opioids . . ." I start running down the list, but Jackie merely pushes me toward the closed door.

"Go check it out yourself and let us know what you think," she says a little too enthusiastically. They nod in unison, encouraging me towards the closed door.

"Okay, okay," I say as I push open the door. The room is a little on the dark side, the curtains closed with only the bathroom light on. "Mr. Washington, my name is Patrice, one of the nurses here at the hospital. I've come to check to see if you need anything."

As I approach the bed, an old, grizzled face peers up at me, the deep furrows around his mouth and eyes attesting to what must be a very hard life.

"What did you say your name was?" he asks, his voice cracking.

"I said my name is Patrice, and . . ."

"Well, young lady, I really don't like your name or the tone of your voice neither. I suggest you leave my room right now."

And with that, the surprising old man has slithered out of bed, IV pole and all, taken me by the elbow and deposited me outside his room, the door closing behind me so fast, I don't know what hit me.

The laughter from the nurses' station spins me around, and I see the conspirators smirking as I walk back toward them, still a bit dazed by how little time it took to be thrown out of Mr. Washington's room.

"Did anyone get the number of that truck?" I ask as I approach them.

They are cackling by the time I finally get it.

"You set me up!" I whisper incredulously. "You set me up! You actually paged me to watch me get thrown out of that man's room!"

Jackie recovers before the others. "I plead guilty," she giggles. "We just needed a laugh this morning. It's been tough up here. We know Mr. Washington from a previous admit. He's a touch paranoid."

"A touch?" I ask sarcastically. "Is this poor man on any medication?"

"He is now," Vernon replies. He lightly punches me in the shoulder. "Gotcha."

I smile, too. I understand the need for a ruse in a place where there is so much suffering. It is an error in judgment to believe that the staff don't suffer, too. I lighten up with them and begin to relax, the laughter a soothing balm for my own raw nerves.

"What else are you doing for him?"

"We got it covered," Vernon says. "He responds better to me, so I'm going to be his primary while he's with us. We're hoping the medication will start to be effective within the next 24 hours or so. I'm checking on him every 15 minutes, but also giving him some space. He's needing to feel safe here first. Don't want to pressure him too fast. We really haven't started his chemo yet—needed him to stabilize on his meds first; otherwise, he'll be thinking we're poisoning him."

"Kind of ironic, wouldn't you say, Vernon?" and I give him a raised eyebrow.

"Yeah, yeah, I know. I guess it depends on your point of view. We've diagnosed him right out of the DSM-IV Revised as G.O.M.S."

"Grumpy Old Man Syndrome?" I ask.

He nods with a grin. "Anyway, if we really need any help with him, we'll be sure to call you. Actually, we've kind of adopted him." They're all still smirking at me.

"I know he's in good hands," I agree, smirking back.

10

AN OLD WOUND STILL FESTERING

As I walk away from the station, I remember Diane's forlorn-looking face waiting out in the hallway. I'm thinking she might still be where I left her since I couldn't have been gone more than a few minutes; I don't see her, however, so I saunter on down the hallway to the other station. She's not there either, and as I look at the board to check out her assigned patients, I don't notice her in any of their rooms. Someone in one of the nearby rooms is having a coughing spell. A moist one from the gurgle of it. Diane swings out of the break room, running into me.

"I was just looking for you. Do you have time to talk now?"

"Sure, why don't we go back in here?" and she heads back to where she came from. The break room on each floor is always a study in caregiver insouciance: waste baskets completely overflowing; a box of stale doughnuts on the table, the jelly congealed on the waxed paper; the microwave door standing open to a mess of cooked-on glop that must be incubating the next strain of antibiotic-resistant organisms; mailboxes stuffed with all sorts of official papers that haven't been rummaged through; and a sign that lamely proclaims, "Your mother doesn't work here. Clean up your own mess."

Diane sits down, her speech immediately pressured.

"It's Mrs. Litweiller," she says grimly, her voice cracking. "I think she's seriously depressed. I can't really seem to reach her."

"What makes you say that?" I ask, sitting down across from her.

"She's just not responding to me when I'm in there working with her. I just can't seem to make a connection. I think she really could use some extra help from you."

There's something about the tone of her voice. I ask more questions.

"Can you give me an example?"

"Well, like before I saw you in the hallway, I was finishing her assessment, and I asked her if she's depressed since her illness has become terminal. And she says to me that no, she's not depressed."

"Sounds like she is responding to you."

"Well, really I think she is minimizing the issue. I think she is just trying to avoid dealing with it. I really feel like she's brushing me off." Diane is swallowing hard. A lot. I notice because I've started swallowing hard with her.

"So it seems implausible to you that she could be at end of life and not really be depressed?"

"Well, when you put it that way, I guess so," she says although she seems a bit confused by the direction the conversation is taking.

By way of explanation, I continue. "You took care of Lilli Chan several months ago, didn't you?" She nods. "Well, I remember Bernardi consulting me on her and asking me to evaluate her for depression because she was demonstrating some of the vegetative signs—you know, lack of appetite, sleep disturbances, and so on." She nods again. "Well, I completed an initial assessment and Dr. Bernardi thought I miscalled it."

"What did you think was going on with her?"

"It appeared to me that Mrs. Chan was dying and was pretty much accepting of it. She told me she was sad to be leaving her family but that at age 87 she couldn't think of anything else she needed to do to complete her life. She wasn't depressed, just slowly dying. People who are dying tend to eat less."

"What did Dr. Bernardi say?"

"Oh, he disagreed with me and put her on an antidepressant anyway."

"Did she get any better?"

"Yeah. She died. Before the antidepressant could become clinically effective."

I smile at the plot twist at the end of my story, but Diane only looks more dismal.

"Well, Mrs. Chan was 87, and Margaret Litweiller is 51. I really need for her to understand what is going on here. I really do think she is in denial."

"*You* really need?" I ask. "What is it that *you* really need, Diane?"

Her professional exterior fails her, and she looks down, shaking her head. "I need her to take this seriously so that she has a chance to do this the right way."

"And what way is that?" I ask gently.

"To be able to have meaningful time with her family, to have time to say good-bye, to plan for how to leave."

"Diane, I am going out on a limb here, but does being with Margaret Litweiller remind you of being with anyone else?"

She looks up in shocked realization. "Yeah, now that you mention it. It reminds me of being with my mother. She died three years ago."

"Let me guess. Metastatic breast cancer," I say.

She nods, beginning to weep.

"And so what happened between you and your mother during her dying?"

She swallows hard. "She couldn't talk about it. Or wouldn't. When we were together, she said she didn't want to dwell on the negative. So we had to pretend it wasn't happening. It was terrible."

"Sounds like you wanted to make contact with her very much, but it just wasn't her way."

"My mother was pretty much like that throughout her life. Always looking at the bright side. I think she really wanted to protect all of us from what was going on. But it just left me feeling lonely."

"Kind of like now?"

"Yeah, I guess. Kind of like now."

Someone I don't recognize walks in to get something out of the refrigerator and puts it into the sorry-looking microwave, beeping the poor thing into submission. He takes one look at us and walks out.

"Sounds like your mother died the way she lived—on her own terms. You supported her choice in how she handled it. What a good daughter you were."

She looks up at me and thanks me, but it is weak and unconvincing.

"And so what do you suppose is happening between you and Mrs. Litweiller here?"

"I'm over-identifying with the situation. What's that called again?"

"You mean counter-transference?"

"Oh, yeah, counter-transference."

"Who's Charge up here today?"

"It's Yvonne," she says, wiping her face with a crumbling tissue.

"Let's go ask Yvonne to change your assignment, and then let's you and I set up a couple of appointments together. What do you think?"

She nods and looks relieved. "You know," I say as we pass the guy going back in to retrieve his food, "the Buddhists say it's easy to keep your heart open in heaven. So much harder to do so in hell."

She looks at me silently and gives me a hug as we move back to the station where Yvonne is speaking with a family member. As Diane and I queue up in line, my pager goes off. I tell Diane I am going to return the page and she can describe the situation to Yvonne, that I'll be right there.

"It's me," I say into the receiver, juggling my calendar and a pen.

"Yeah, it's T.J. down in outpatient chemo. We've got a little problem down here. Are you freed up to stop by?"

"What kind of little problem?" I ask.

"Well, this patient is here for her first treatment and everything is going swimmingly except that when I insert the IV needle, everything went south."

I see Diane approach Yvonne and point to where I'm standing in the station. Yvonne nods in my direction and keeps on listening to Diane.

"So what do you mean, everything went south?"

"Everything. Her voice, her expression, I mean I don't know what the heck I'm looking at here."

"Well, I hope I have an answer for you. Give me ten minutes, can you?"

"We're not going anywhere down here, but it is freaking us all out."

I hang up the phone and approach Yvonne. Diane has already left.

"Are you cool with that?" I ask her. Yvonne is erasing her assignment sheet and her cell phone is ringing.

"I'm just going to switch her with Sylvia. They've both had each other's patients, so the patients won't know anything is up. I'm glad she talked to someone about it. She seemed a little stressed out today, but I didn't know where it was coming from."

Someone else is waiting in line behind me to talk to Yvonne, so I am feeling pressed to move on. "No problem," I tell her. "I'm glad you were able to work it out."

"So am I," she says. "It's not always that easy."

She is right. Being charge nurse means having to make everybody happy—patients, families, staff, management. Decisions need to be made quickly, competently, and economically for at least 8 hours straight.

I'm back down the stairway again, grateful for the opportunity to be alone. Rather than racing to the next floor, I slow down deliberately to give myself a bit of time to catch up.

11

BETSY AND ELIZABETH

I know something is afoot in the outpatient chemo clinic when I find most of the staff in the report room.

"Gosh, who's with the patients?" I ask. I'm joking. Kind of.

"Well, we're a little spooked, it's true," Donetta replies. "Mary Margaret is in there with her right now." As she speaks, a long, low wail sounds from down the hall.

"So what's that?"

"Well, it was the funniest thing," T.J. says as he twirls a set of keys around his index finger. "I showed her into the treatment room, explained the set-up, the drill, oriented her to the whole process, and she was just fine."

"Okay, slow down and tell me who we are talking about here," I say, reaching for a chair and pulling it out to sit at a table strewn with half-completed charts, an assignment sheet, and a pile of forgettable-looking hospital memoranda.

T.J. pulls up a chair as well. "This is the first treatment for Elizabeth Pagura, 38-year-old patient of Dr.

Schoen. She's being treated for lung cancer. Anyway, she seems like a nice enough person and all, a little anxious, but nothing terrible for a first chemo treatment. Anyway, she sits in the chair, and she's got some sort of professional journal with her to read, and a coffee, and anyway, I'm telling her what to expect before I do anything to her. I warm her veins and bring in the IV lines and bag, and I start hunting for a vein. She starts looking a little green behind the gills, and she breaks out into this cold sweat as I stick her." As he's talking, T.J.'s voice becomes more pressured, and he looks a bit unnerved as he continues. "And all of a sudden, she lets out this real high scream. Nearly freaked me out. I stop what I'm doing and before I know it, she's thrown her glasses across the room and is on the floor in the corner in a fetal position."

"Sounds pretty extreme," I agree.

"You haven't heard the half of it," he says. "So I put all the IV equipment inside the cabinet and try to talk her down. I even get on the floor with her, trying to calm her. And as I get closer to her, she starts talking like she's a kid—in a kid's voice. And I swear I'm not kidding when I tell you that when we started the whole thing off, her eyes were big and brown. By the time I get on the floor with her, her eyes are green. It's the damndest thing I ever saw. I mean, I have heard of stress, but this is over the top." T.J. is clearly rattled.

"So what's going on in there right now?" I ask.

"Well, we couldn't leave her alone while we waited for you, but she seems terrified of us. Mary Margaret is in there with her holding down the fort."

God bless Mary Margaret, a seasoned veteran.

Before we can move, another wail comes from down the hall. As I walk out the door, other patients in the area look warily down the hallway.

"Donetta, see what you can do about getting these patients into treatment rooms or back into the waiting room out front. I don't want them freaked out, too," I say.

She nods and begins to corral people out of the hallways like a sheep dog working a flock. There's no surprise as to where Elizabeth's room is. By the time I come close enough, I can hear a low-pitch keening coming from inside. I stand outside the door and wonder what I'm going to find on the other side once I open it.

Mary Margaret is seated on the floor in front of a pile of clothes. She looks relieved to see me and jerks her head over to the clothing. There, within the clothing, is a shrunken little lump of a human being. In fact, if I didn't know any better, I would say it is a child. Elizabeth Pagura is shivering and weeping in the corner, waves of fear washing off her so palpable, they're hitting me, too. My heart goes out to her immediately although there is no doubt that the situation is really daunting. For all of us.

"I'll take it from here, Mary Margaret," I whisper, and she nods as she indicates she will be right outside the door in case I need her.

As the door closes behind her, I take a seat on the stool in front of it to let Elizabeth get used to the new presence. Her brown hair haloes her head in ringlets that seem to spring in all directions. When she looks up long enough to inspect me, I can see that whatever make-up she walked in with is now smeared all over her face, giving her the appearance of a fugitive from a *What Ever Happened to Baby Jane* movie set. I take a long, deep breath.

"My name is Patrice. What's your name?" I ask simply.

She doesn't look up, keeping her face cupped in her hands. "Betsy," she whimpers.

"I like that name," I say softly. I let that sit awhile, deciding to pick my way through the landmines slowly, trying to gingerly sift through whatever she is willing to share with me without pressuring her to do so. If I am not careful, we will be back to square one immediately. And often. On a hunch, I ask, "How old are you, Betsy?"

She holds up four fingers without looking up.

"Such a big girl, and you are here all alone. Didn't anyone come with you today?"

She lets out a deep sigh.

"It must be very scary to be in such a big place by yourself. Who usually looks after you?"

"Elizabeth usually takes care of these things for us," comes the whispered response. A thumb quickly pokes into her lipstick-smeared mouth.

"Where is Elizabeth now?" I ask tentatively, trying not to move too fast too quickly.

"Oh, she's around," the small voice replies. "It's just that when that man brought out all the needles, I really got scared, and Elizabeth couldn't keep me from getting out. I hate needles. They remind me of things."

"What kind of things, Betsy?"

She quickly turns away from me and vigorously sucks her thumb. I am going too fast here. I need to have time for us to regroup.

"Say, are you hungry or thirsty? Would you like something to eat?"

"Whaddya got?" she asks without turning around. She's twisting a strand of run-away hair around a finger of the other hand.

"Well, we have ice cream and Popsicles."

"Do you have grape Popsicles?" she asks turning quickly, her green eyes big, thumb hovering in the air.

"I believe we do, Betsy."

"Well, I'll take one of those if you have one."

"Coming right up." I open the door a tad and ask Mary Margaret to retrieve a Popsicle. I happen to notice a stethoscope on the side table as I shut the door again.

"While we are waiting," I try guardedly, "would you like to listen to your heart beat?"

"What's that thing?"

I show her how I put it in my ears and how I can listen to my own heartbeat.

"Can I listen?" she asks.

"Sure, come on over," I say, offering her the stethoscope.

Suddenly curious, she walks on her hands and knees over to where I am sitting and this kid in the grown woman's body allows me to fit her ears with the stethoscope. She looks at me in awe as the lub-dub of my heart registers in her ears.

"Now my turn," she says, and she moves the instrument to her own chest. She allows me to place it for her where she can hear her own heart.

"Wow!" Her smile is innocent yet a bit off-kilter. One does not expect to see such an expression of awe on the face of an adult. That's a bit unfortunate, I think to myself.

Just then, there is a quiet knock at the door. I reach back behind me to turn the doorknob. A grape Popsicle is thrust in my face, and I thank Mary Margaret for responding so quickly. As I peel back the paper, Betsy reaches for it and politely thanks me. As she licks it, the purple of the Popsicle collides with the lipstick. She seems to relax with each slurp, the stethoscope still dangling from her ears. Worlds collide.

As I remove the stethoscope and hand her a paper towel to catch the drippings, I ask her, "Better now?"

She nods.

"So tell me Betsy, does Elizabeth see anybody special for the problems you both have with things that scare you?"

"Like who?"

"Oh, I don't know, a special doctor or nurse who gives you medicine to help you feel better when things get scary? Who talks to you about the scary things?"

"Elizabeth takes care of those things for us."

"Any chance I can talk to Elizabeth right now?'

"Can I keep the Popsicle?"

"Of course you can, honey."

"Well, okay then."

And just like that, suddenly, big brown eyes are staring back at me, frowning at the grape Popsicle dripping down her sleeve.

"Where did this come from?" Elizabeth asks. "And who are you?"

She hands the dripping flavored ice to me, and I reintroduce myself. She gets off the floor, blotting her clothes with the paper towels, looking sheepish. She squints as she happens to catch a glimpse of herself in the mirror hanging over the sink and groans as she tries to mend her face.

"Where are my glasses?" she asks.

"Elizabeth?" I ask guardedly as I hand them to her.

"Yes, I'm back," she says turning around, sweeping her hair back away from her face. "I suppose this means you have just met Betsy," she says pointing to the melting Popsicle.

"Yes. Are you all right now?"

"I'm fine. I guess I should have asked someone else to come with me when my sister came down with the flu."

"Elizabeth, I'm going to recommend that we don't start your chemo today. Is that all right?"

"I really wish we could though. I just want to get this going, and get it over with as soon as possible."

"Does Dr. Schoen know you have a multiple personality disorder?"

"I'm not sure really. He can see I'm on all this medication, but I guess we were just so focused on the cancer, we forgot about Betsy."

"Well, Betsy sure got scared. Can you tell me what she is scared of?"

Elizabeth takes a big deep sigh. "I really don't want to go into the details here, but I'm a childhood incest survivor. I see Dr. Karen Hooks for this and have been on medication for years."

"Did you or Dr. Hooks discuss that your treatment might trigger your condition? I'm sure she must have known that needles would have been involved in the chemotherapy. It might be wise to consider readjusting the dosage of your medication to compensate for the extra stress burden you are under right now."

Elizabeth starts looking a little pasty, and I'm afraid I'm going to lose her again, so I say quickly.

"Elizabeth, let's talk to Dr. Schoen about rescheduling this, and then set up a meeting with Dr. Hooks to determine how we can proceed so that we can safely treat you without pre-disposing you to dissociate."

She looks relieved and disappointed at the same time. "You know, I really thought I could handle this on my own," she muses, matter-of-factly. "I guess I couldn't." She licks more of the grape Popsicle goo off her fingers.

"You know, Elizabeth, folks who don't have the challenges you face have a rough time with this, too, so please don't judge yourself so harshly."

She nods peremptorily.

I call Mary Margaret back in. She sticks her head in the door and peers curiously around the corner at Elizabeth.

"Mary Margaret, can you inform Elizabeth's oncologist that she has multiple personality disorder and we're recommending that her treatment today be deferred until we can check with her psychiatrist as to how to safely proceed?"

Mary Margaret looks back at Elizabeth. "I am so sorry we didn't know about this in advance. We could have been better prepared. We'll do better next time. I promise."

Talk about the right thing to say, I think to myself. I am also thinking I probably need to do an in-service for the out-patient chemotherapy staff to prepare them for her next appointment. And anyone else like her who might come walking in through the door.

"Elizabeth, when I go back to my office, I'm going to call Dr. Schoen, too, and with your written permission, I'm going to call Dr. Hooks, so we can get a plan together, okay?"

She nods as I hand her a release of information sheet to sign and write the psychiatrist's phone number from her card on my clinical note sheet, which I stick back into my over-stuffed pocket.

"Mary Margaret, how long will it take to get Elizabeth re-scheduled?"

"Probably just a few days."

"Will that work out okay?"

Elizabeth nods.

"Do you think we can set up a time to meet together before your next chemo appointment?"

"I think that would probably be a good idea," Elizabeth agrees.

"I'll call you with an appointment time as soon as I talk to your doctors then. Mary Margaret will make sure you get another chemo appointment. Oh, and Elizabeth?"

She looks back at me, glasses back on her face, brown eyes staring at me quizzically.

"Here's another Popsicle for the road. For Betsy."

She smiles, takes the Popsicle, and turns down the corridor following Mary Margaret.

I sit there for a moment, wondering where I was in my day before I met up with Betsy. I feel myself zoning out a bit and realize I'm a bit on overload with everyone else's crises. And that's when the pager screams in my pocket.

12

Sleeping Beauty Awakens

"This is Patrice."

"Hi, this is Li Chan. I'm a nurse in the surgical intensive care unit, and we have a situation here. I was told you might be able to help us out with it."

"Sure, Li. Is it one of our patients?"

"Well, actually not. It would probably be easier to talk to you about this face to face. Do you have some time today for us to get together?"

"Is now okay?" I ask tentatively. "I'm just finishing up something here. Do you want me to meet you over there?"

"It would be great if you could," she responds appreciatively.

"Sure, give me 10 minutes."

If it doesn't have to do with one of our patients, I have to wonder what the mystery is all about. Her call has certainly piqued my curiosity. Many of our oncology patients are admitted directly into the surgical intensive care unit post-operatively, so I am familiar with the unit. It is unusual for me to get a call unless it is about one of our patients or families.

Entering into the SICU is tantamount to accessing a hospital's inner sanctum. There is a different rhythm here, a vibration that hums to all the mechanical paraphernalia to which humans can be hooked up—so much so that the humans often take on the appearance, if not the identity, of cyborgs. As I pass by individual cubicles that double as rooms, caregivers are typically monitoring machinery, the person in the bed often seeming superfluous.

Li meets me at the door of the nurses' conference room and thanks me for coming over. She is young and soft-spoken. There is also a resident and a medical student in attendance. They introduce themselves peremptorily to me and invite me to sit down.

"Thanks for coming over," Li begins. "Here is our situation. About a month ago, one of our patients, Richard Stultz, a 21-year-old patient of Dr. Volakis, had what was thought to be a routine arthroscopic knee repair. He tore some ligaments during a soccer game. At any rate, it wasn't long afterward that it became apparent that the knee was infected, but the infection was so virulent, the patient became septic quickly."

"Happened that quickly?"

"Yeah, it happened to be an antibiotic-resistant organism and it took awhile to get on top of it."

"What happened?"

The resident took up the narrative. "Well, the patient actually became unconscious and has remained so for the past month."

"What's his prognosis?" I ask, the mother in me worried already. This could happen to anybody's kid. It already has once today.

"Well, actually quite good. Now," the resident replies guardedly.

"But?" I prompt.

Li continues. "Here's the thing. Richard is beginning to come out of the coma, and the infection is completely gone. He should make a full recovery. The only problem is that in order to save him from the septicemia, a decision was made to do an above the knee amputation."

They are all looking at me meaningfully as I finally grasp what they are telling me.

"So you are saying that the last thing this kid remembers is that he was going under to have a knee repair done and he is waking up to find . . ." I cannot even finish putting it into words.

The resident nods. "He will have no idea what he's been through. That he has almost died, that he has lost his leg. He is waking up thinking that his knee has been repaired and that with a little rehab, he will be back on the soccer field."

I stare at them, and they stare back. My eyes fill up with tears for this kid. The medical student's leg is bouncing up and down so nervously it rocks the table a bit. He's probably not much older than the patient.

The resident brushes his honey blond hair off his face with both hands as he leans back in his chair. "So the reason we brought you in on this," he continues, "is that we understand you work with patients around body image issues and we thought perhaps you could help us with Richard."

Everyone in the room is younger than me and probably over-identifying with Richard. It is a daunting challenge. How to tell someone this kind of news. I take a deep breath.

"So, okay, tell me where he's at, consciousness-wise. What are we talking about here? Now. Today."

"He is waking up," Li says. "We have him on a PCA pump to help us address the phantom pain situation. The stump itself is healing well. But his only therapy has been passive range of motion." Her voice trails off.

"Obviously," I agree, returning their stares. "So my role here is to introduce him to the idea that he is without his leg now." This is not a question.

They are all three nodding.

"Does he have family?"

"His parents live in North Carolina. We've called them, and they are flying back in. They just went back several days ago to pay bills, check the house."

"So when do you want me to start?"

They all look at me.

"Do you have time right now?"

They walk me to Richard's room. I take a big breath outside and once again pray that somehow I will know what to say, what to do, when I cross the threshold. As I do, I take in the scene. Richard is a good-looking young man despite what he has been through. He is connected to a variety of drips and telemonitoring devices that give his appearance that strange cyborg quality. It is at once disturbing and reassuring that machines can stand in for our organ systems until we can stand on our own two feet. Or one foot.

I approach his bed, noticing that the others have vanished already. I guess I am on my own here. No one to even introduce me. But then again, I remember that Richard probably doesn't even know who they are either. I have to keep in mind that he is existing in a time warp and that as he awakens, he will have lost the month that everyone else has had, that he is a whole month behind the rest of us.

His brown lashes flicker, and he stirs in bed. Some moaning. I am mindful that his patient controlled analgesia will now have to be recalibrated based on his conscious, verbal indications of his pain rating, and not just the staff's assessment of pain levels from his nonverbal behavior. My, oh my.

I touch his hand softly. "Richard."

His eyes flutter open, and he tries to focus on my face but is unsuccessful. He mutters something that sounds like "Give me a chance," but I can't be sure.

He is licking lips that are dried and parched looking. I find a swab, moisten it in some cold water, and swab out his mouth. I wipe his face with a moist, tepid washcloth.

He grimaces a bit and makes another effort to open his eyes, this time a little more successfully. He looks up at me with brown eyes that have not seen the light of day in a month.

"I didn't think it would hurt this bad," he groans.

I reach over and ring the call button. "I'll get you some extra medicine, Richard."

He nods as though he comprehends, but I can't be sure. In a matter of minutes, Li enters the cubicle, and I explain that before we can do anything Richard will need better pain relief. She nods and promises to return shortly. When she does, she reprograms his pain pump and gives him a hefty bolus of morphine. Within minutes, his face is a bit more relaxed and he releases the vice grip on my hand.

"Better?"

He nods imperceptibly and starts breathing more deeply. Rather than falling asleep under the influence of the drug, it has the opposite effect, and the relief from the pain for the time being seems to help him come to. He opens those eyes and now is able to sustain a quizzical look right at me.

"I'm still in the hospital, right?"

"Yes. You are still in the hospital."

"Did everything go all right?" he asks, rubbing his face with his pale hands.

"Well, there were some complications, Richard."

"And you are?"

"My name is Patrice. I am one of the clinical nurse specialists here at the hospital."

He refocuses, forehead furrowed. "Complications? What kind of complications?"

I am aware once again of this moment as a turning point in this person's life. I am aware that from now on, he will remember life as before this moment and after this moment. I am aware.

"This will be a lot to absorb, Richard, so I'm going to take it slowly."

I feel him tensing as he understands I am trying to prepare him to receive bad news. It amazes me that this sleeping beauty who was unconscious just yesterday is now awake enough to hear what I am about to say, although I am sure he will need to have it repeated again.

"The surgery itself went well. However, afterwards you developed a serious infection in the operative site. A really severe infection, Richard."

"Is that why it hurts so much?"

"Well, there's more to it than that. The infection was so serious that it spread into your bloodstream very rapidly. So rapidly that you developed a systemic infection. What we call a septicemia."

He is staring at me intently and swallows hard. He is understanding there is more. "Go on," he murmurs quietly.

"Shortly after you developed the systemic infection, you lost consciousness. You were really very, very sick, Richard. So sick, you had to be brought here into the intensive care unit and put on life support."

His eyes widen, and it seems that this is the first opportunity he has taken to actually look around his surroundings.

He seems to grasp now that all the machinery and equipment is not "standard" hospital room issue.

"Are you telling me that I was so sick that I could have died?"

I nod. He puts his hand to his forehead and stares up into the ceiling. "My parents? Are they okay? Are they here?"

"Actually they have been here for quite some time. They just went home to check on things, but now that you are waking up, they are on their way back."

"This must have freaked them out," he says, still absorbing what he is hearing. I let him sit with this for awhile.

"There's more, Richard."

He looks back at me, stricken, as though what I have told him isn't bad enough.

"What else?"

I take a deep breath. "Well, the antibiotics were not holding the infection very well. And there was some sincere thought that if something more serious wasn't done for you, that you wouldn't make it."

"So, what could be done any further than putting me on life support . . ." He stops in mid-sentence, looks down at the bed, and then gropes a hand to where his leg should have been.

"Oh my God, you didn't." He lifts up the covers and peers beneath. He drops the covers, his face contorted into a grimace. "Oh my God, oh my God, oh my God," he sobs. "You didn't, you didn't, you didn't. . ." His voice trails off. If there is a mask for the human emotion of anguish, he is wearing it now.

I stay at the bedside while he sobs and sobs and sobs. There is nothing to say, nothing to do but be with him. Two strangers, one of them bearing witness to the other's suffering. The bed shakes with his sobbing. It is deep-felt. It is mournful. It is soul-wrenching. To help me bear his pain, I must remind myself to breathe.

After awhile he simply closes his eyes and falls back to sleep, whether due to shock, exhaustion, the pain medication, or merely to escape the reality to which he has awakened. I wait to make sure that he is truly out and then quietly withdraw. It is a lot to have had to absorb all at once. And it is definitely not over.

I make my way slowly back to the conference room where Li is charting. She looks up expectantly as I enter, and I sit down across from her.

"You look terrible," she says to me.

"Do I?" I ask. "I guess it's hard to be the messenger."

She nods sympathetically and pours me a cup of water from a pitcher on the table. I take it gratefully, not realizing how thirsty I am.

"Well, he knows, but then he went right out. You know, I'll be needing to come back to help him work through all this."

"We would appreciate it if you would. He's going to need to start rehab here soon, and he'll need to get into some kind of shape to do that. Psychologically speaking."

I nod as I begin looking ahead. "I have a book with narratives and pictures of others who have had amputations who go on to live full lives. I'll bring that back with me when I come back tomorrow."

"Thank you."

"How long is he going to stay here, Li?"

"Once we can make sure he's stable, he'll probably be transferred over to rehab as soon as possible."

"Can you all make sure that his pain management program is top notch before he gets there? I'd imagine the phantom pain and all those attendant sensations will be very difficult for him if he is expected to work hard in therapy."

"Goes without saying," she agrees. She looks at me sympathetically. "We know this is not your unit, but we appreciate your help with this one. We were feeling a little over our heads in terms of helping him wake up to all this."

"Of course," I say, feeling like the stuffing has just been knocked out of me. And I'm just the messenger.

And that's when the pager goes off.

13

SHE WHO DOTH PROTEST TOO MUCH

It's Marvelle again.

"What's up?" I ask, feeling myself already begin to steel myself.

"You remember Tamara Salerno? The gal with the abdominal tumor who said she didn't want a colostomy?"

"Yes."

"Well, she drove herself here, more than a two-hour drive, to get here by 9 a.m. for her scheduled surgery. She was bumped off the schedule due to an emergency surgery, and she is fit to be tied. I think she's going to walk."

"As in have her surgery rescheduled?"

"No, as in walk away and not come back."

"Have you notified her surgeon?"

"He's tied up in that emergency surgery."

"Okay, I guess I'll be right down then."

"I don't know if I can keep her down here until you can get here."

"I'm on my way, Marvelle. Sit on her if you have to."

By the time I get down to the lobby, I spot Marvelle standing between Tamara and the exit door. It looks like a Mexican stand-off. I am wondering whether there is anything we can do to induce her to stay at this point.

Marvelle looks relieved when she sees me, her reinforcement, approach from behind Tamara. I have no idea what I am going to say or do next.

"Tamara, you remember Patrice, don't you?" she remarks gesturing towards me.

Tamara spins around and faces me squarely.

"Listen, there is absolutely no way I am going to let any of you people touch me now," she hisses. People passing by in the lobby look at our little tableau and immediately begin to steer clear of us as we block one of the doorways.

"I can see how upset you are, Tamara. Anybody would be upset."

"Now don't 'manage' me," she warns me off. "I won't be patronized. I told you I didn't want this thing to begin with. Now I drive down here and spend three hours—*three hours*—waiting for you all to get your act together and do your jobs. Do you know how long I've been without food and water?"

"I really am so sorry about all of this, truly. If that emergency were you, wouldn't you want your doctor to have seen to you immediately?"

"But I am an emergency!"

Not only is she furious, she is also frightening other people walking through the lobby, leaving me to figure out how to do some sort of damage control when an elderly woman in a wheelchair tries to come through the door we are blocking.

"Let's go somewhere where we aren't blocking other people getting into the hospital," I suggest, guiding her ever so gently by the arm across the lobby toward an unoccupied room. I can see that she is feeling badly about the woman in the wheelchair. Marvelle follows at a discreet distance, wanting to make sure her lobby is once more returned to a non-combat zone.

As I close the door behind us, I see that Tamara is unable to settle down and is pacing around the small room like a caged animal. I sit down in front of the door and wait her out, aware of the agitated energy that is quickly suffocating the room.

"I am sick and tired of all of this," she spits. "The cancer is bad enough! But to be treated like a leper like this is just more than I can take!"

I decide not to defend the hospital, or the patient who apparently took an emergent turn for the worse, thereby bumping Tamara from the schedule for the time being. I watch her pace back and forth and try to remember to breathe deeply, hoping that my rhythm will become contagious to her and not the other way around.

"I drive up here all by myself. You know what time I had to leave the house this morning just to get here on time, so you people could carve me up? Do you know I haven't had a thing to eat or drink since yesterday? And all for what?"

I watch her retrace her steps over and over. Is it just wishful thinking on my part, or is she starting to wind down a bit? She may be wearing herself out. I just keep watching her.

"When does this nightmare ever end?! When do I finally get to wake up and get on with my life?" She stops in front of me and looks at me as if I could actually have an answer for her.

"Anybody would be angry in your situation," I say as softly as possible. "Certainly you don't have to like it. I am so very sorry, Tamara, that you have to go through all of this. I'm so very sorry."

And with that, she begins a deep weeping that breaks my heart. She stands forlornly in the middle of the room, head hanging in her hands, her hair hiding her face. Her wail is the wail of every human who has ever suffered and who feels alone in it. I rise quietly and approach her. Gently; I put my arms around her, and she lets me rock her softly back and forth, back and forth, back and forth. We rock until her breathing matches the rhythm of the rocking. And then we slowly stop.

She cannot look up at me and seems embarrassed by the unabashed flow of mucus dripping from her face. I grab for the tissues and hand them to her while she sheepishly mops up. All the power she felt when she was angry has been dissipated, and she is now left feeling vulnerable. She collapses on the couch, tissues to her nose. The effort to escape her powerlessness through her rage has left her humbled, exhausted. I am exhausted with her, and I have only watched.

I sit down when it seems she is more composed. Her whimpering resembles that of a small child—the Sturm und Drang rage against an unjust universe. Big whimpers as she strives to catch her breath.

"I don't know how much longer I can go on," she whispers.

"As long as it takes," I say simply.

"I feel like a big baby. You must think I'm an idiot." She wipes at her face, smoothing back her hair, unable to make eye contact.

"Actually, being with you makes me think of a poem I once read about strong women. Something to the effect that as they clean out the cesspools of the world, they cry, that with every birthed baby, they lose another tooth. Being courageous isn't pretty, after all."

"Who said anything about being courageous?"

"I think courage isn't about looking like Grace Kelley as we walk into the lion's den. It's about being stinking afraid and walking in there anyway."

"Well, if that's your definition, then I must get the Cowardly Lion award." She smiles dimly, looking up at me under a tussle of her wet bangs.

I smile back at her. "You're in good company. The world is full of Cowardly Lions. Tears don't just happen to babies, you know. They happen to all of us. It's not that you're a baby, Tamara. You're simply human."

She absorbs this without saying anything. We just sit there for awhile, each of us lost in our own thoughts, each of us waiting separately, yet together, our breathing in synch now.

I don't really know how long we are waiting when there is a soft knock on the door, and it opens slowly. Marvelle sticks her head in the door cautiously to check on us.

"The surgeon called down to say that you should report up to pre-op in 15 minutes."

"You mean they are still going to take me today?" Tamara asks surprised.

"Of course," Marvelle replies. "You don't think he would leave you hanging like this, do you? The other patient had a fistula that blew and required a rapid repair. You're up next."

Tamara breaks out in a full smile. "Ironic, isn't it?" she asks. "I'm relieved you're going to do the surgery on me that I said I didn't want. I guess thinking I wasn't going to get it left me feeling deprived."

Marvelle smiles back at her. I can tell she is relieved that Tamara has had a change of heart. She gives me a meaningful look and then closes the door behind her.

"I suppose I must look awful," Tamara demures, her present self-consciousness a stark contrast to her demeanor of just an hour ago.

"I think you look beautiful," I say. And I really mean it.

She looks at me gratefully, sensing my sincerity, hugs me, and goes to the door, turning to say, "I'm going to the rest room to clean up. Thanks, I mean it. Thanks."

I nod. "Would you like some company up to pre-op?"

"What? Afraid I'm going to run?"

"Not now," I say. And I mean it.

"Naw, I'm okay. Really—I'm okay now."

I believe her. "Would it be okay with you if I checked up on you tomorrow?"

"I would be disappointed if you didn't." She looks at me levelly and closes the door behind herself.

Now there goes some kind of woman, I think, sighing loudly. I must have been holding my breath, unaware.

And with that, the pager goes off. It's Marvelle again.

14

AN UNANTICIPATED MESSAGE

"Your appointment just walked in."

"Can I use this room for her?" I ask.

"I'll send her right back. By the way, everything okay in there?"

"Yeah, she's on her way up. Say, would you do me a favor, and tell everyone else out there to hold all their emergencies until tomorrow?"

"Yeah. I'll get right on it," she says dryly. The door opens, and Marilyn Rubin sticks her head in the door.

"Are you ready for me?" she asks, a quick smile on her face. I am unabashedly relieved that the next person I have to deal with isn't initially hostile, waking up from a coma, or in a fugue state.

"Yes, come on in, Marilyn. Do you mind if we leave the door open for a little bit before we get started?" The air still feels dense with Tamara's intense emotionality. If I had a sage stick, I'd smudge the room of her pain before getting started. Marilyn, however, is all business and swings off her jacket and throws it over the couch as she sinks down next to it.

"What do you want to work on today?" I ask, taking my seat again.

"Well, you know, I am not really convinced that the treatment my doctor wants to put me through here is really in my best interest. I would like to explore more complementary and alternative therapies, really. And then if they don't work, try the more extreme conventional treatment."

Marilyn's tumor is aggressive, huge, and unrelenting. The doctors have proposed a course of industrial strength chemotherapy first to try to shrink it, then surgery, to be followed up with more chemotherapy and even radiation. The plan is for her to get the whole megillah, and she knows it.

"Well, you know, Marilyn, I think you use the best of what complementary and alternative medicine offers and combine it with the best of conventional medicine and develop your own customized treatment program. Not one or the other, but both combined together makes for a very strong program."

Marilyn is ready for this. "Yes, I know, but I don't want all that poison, mutilation, and burning to healthy tissue." She knows I can't argue the merits of that. "I think I should be building up my immune system instead of tearing it down, especially now." Again, can't argue with that. In 50 years, I believe people will look back on conventional cancer treatments and shake their heads at the medieval barbarity of it all. But we're not 50 years from now, however, and I know how virulent her tumor is. I take another tack.

"I know you have done all your homework, have read all your labs, reports, scans. This really isn't about logic because you have had access to all that information already. I'd like to suggest we do some more guided imagery together. Just to see what other alogical information we can tap into to help with your decision making."

"I'm open to that," she says with a shrug. "I've got nothing to lose."

"Well, great, then. You know the drill."

I close the door as she gets herself into a comfortable position on the couch, works the knots out of her neck, removes her glasses, and folds her hands on her lap.

"Ready?"

She nods and closes her eyes; and then I begin.

"Take a nice deep breath. This is the signal breath, the signal to the rest of your body that we are entering into a special time and place set aside just for you. All subsequent breaths will be breathed normally, rhythmically and peacefully. In and out, in and out, in and out. You will be hearing sounds from inside the room, sounds from outside the room. Nothing to change, nothing to judge, just letting your awareness move from one sound to the next."*

Marilyn, from having had previous experiences with this modality, is already deeply relaxed, her facial muscles soft, her breath long and languid.

I continue. "You'll be having thoughts about what's happened in the past, what's happening now, and what's going to happen in the future. I would like you to detach yourself from your thoughts, and project them up onto a movie screen in your imagination. Nothing to change, nothing to judge. Just watching them come and go as if they have a life of their

*This exercise is based on Piero Ferrucci's *What We May Be, Techniques for Psychological and Spiritual Growth*, Tarcher Penguin, NY, 1983.

own. Because right now all you have to do is breathe. And as you continue to breathe, you allow your body to become an empty vessel, and let your breath breathe you."

Marilyn's posture is slack. She is such a quick study, I think.

"You find yourself in a lovely spring meadow. The air is fresh with the fragrance of new things in bloom, the breeze invigorating yet warm with the sun, which kisses you on the very top of your head. You hear the sounds of insects humming nearby, birds calling to one another. You look around and note at least a hundred different shades of green. You breathe in, you breathe out."

And she does.

"As you continue breathing, you allow the issues that surround your cancer treatment decision to become formulated into questions. Questions that will be asked later. Allow a few moments for these concerns to be articulated in your imagination."

Marilyn is a study in relaxed concentration. I am thinking it would be very easy for her to move into this exercise with foregone conclusions. As usual, I am always curious as to what people will come up with when bridged to their own inner wisdom. What kind of picture they paint when handed their own canvas, brushes, and pigments. A subtle shift in Marilyn's energy level cues me that I can move on.

"It is such a beautiful day that you decide to take a journey, a journey from the meadow to the foot of a nearby mountain. There is a path not far from where you are standing that leads you there, and you find yourself taking your questions with you and embarking on your journey. Little by little, you approach the foot of the mountain. And it is such a fine day, that you decide spontaneously to ascend the mountain, and you do so now."

The change in Marilyn's breathing indicates she is indeed climbing.

"With every step, you feel lighter, more invigorated, more energized. The terrain begins to change. The flora and fauna begin to change. You continue your ascent, ever higher, ever higher. Until gradually and eventually, you spot a cloud up ahead that hangs halfway around the mountain. You are sure footed, and the path is well-marked. Despite the misting, you continue to make your way up and up and up, despite the vapor of the cloud. In fact, you find the cooling mist refreshing as you continue your ascent. Eventually you emerge from on top of the cloud and can hardly believe how crystalline clear the air is up here. You continue climbing so that gradually and eventually you spot the summit of the mountain up ahead of you, the very peak. And once you make that peak, you take a nice deep breath."

And Marilyn does.

"As you continue to breathe, look around in a 360-degree circle, taking in the big picture, but also noticing that even the details come into high resolution. Notice how clearly you can see from this vantage point. Allow yourself to absorb the peace that comes with being on the mountain top."

Indeed, Marilyn looks peaceful. I give her a chance to soak in it for a bit before proceeding.

"After awhile, you become aware that you are not alone up on the mountain top. You become aware of a wise presence dwelling up there. You decide that since it is such a glorious day, you will invite the wise presence to be with you. Allow the first image that comes to mind to represent this wise presence. And when you have the wise presence with you, you take another deep breath."

Marilyn breathes deeply almost immediately, a little smile playing at her lips.

"As you spend time with the wise presence, become aware of the relentless compassion and infinite wisdom available to you. And when you are ready, pose the questions you formulated down in the field to the wise presence. Be open to whatever guidance the wise presence has for you with regard to your questions. You will have five minutes of clock time, which is all the time you will need for this exchange. I will let you know when the time is over."

I watch Marilyn's face carefully. The nonverbal behavior during this part of the exercise is often subtle but also can be very marked. I think the reason I love my work with people so much is that I never know what's coming next. Makes life interesting.

And that is when I notice the tear traveling down Marilyn's left cheek, and another, and another. She looks a bit surprised as if having been kissed awake, not by the handsome prince, but by the ugly toad. And God knows, we all have enough of those.

She sits with the tears silently, her jaw working a bit, brushing the wet away occasionally. But certainly not backing away from any of it. It is what it is, and she is working through it. God love her. I am curious as to what it's all about and decide to not interrupt whatever is going on for her. Time will tell.

Minutes later, I say, "We are nearing the end of the time for the exchange. Finish up whatever feels left undone. When you are ready, thank the wise presence for the guidance you received today and bid the wise presence farewell for now, knowing you can return to the mountain top to consult again when you wish and that you take that power with you everywhere you go."

Marilyn takes a deep breath. The tears seem to have stopped.

"Take another look around you and inhale deeply the peacefulness of the mountain. You decide it is time to return back down the mountain and take the wisdom you have received back to your meadow, back into your normal waking reality. And with the next breath, you begin your descent, noticing each step brings you more energy, more lightness than the last. You continue down, down, down. Until you once again spot the cloud that hangs halfway between the top of the mountain and the bottom. But from the previous experience, you know you can trust yourself and the path, and so you proceed with confidence through the swirling mists until once again you re-emerge from beneath the cloud, continuing your descent. As you do so, the terrain changes, the wildlife changes, and very gradually, very eventually, you find yourself once again on the path that leads from the foot of the mountain back into the meadow."

Marilyn appears composed, if not comforted, by this time.

"And so you complete the last leg of your journey by walking the path back into the meadow, back into the very spot from where you started. You turn around to once again spot your mountain, knowing you can return any time you wish. You look around your meadow and realize you can return here any time you wish as well. You consider the wisdom received from the wise presence and realize it is time to bring it back with you into the here and now. Into this time and space. And you do so, gradually and eventually, by pouring yourself into the body that sits on this couch. Once you are completely here, you can stretch and open your eyes whenever you are ready."

It takes awhile before Marilyn does so. Makes me wonder whether it is because she doesn't want to face what the tears are all about or whether it is because the peacefulness of the meadow is so seductive. Either way, I notice the reluctance to come back to the here and now.

When she does, she sits there looking at me for some time. We all of us have to face our demons, and apparently the exercise has forced Marilyn to face hers.

"Well, that was unexpected," she finally says, rising to pop a tissue out of the nearly empty box.

"How so?" I prompt.

"The wise presence was my mother. My mother, who died of this same cancer when she was my age."

She shakes her head, absently shredding the used tissues as she speaks. "Yeah, at first, I was really elated to see her. I mean I really felt her here." She points to her heart.

"I'm glad you had such a vivid experience."

"Well that is what makes the whole thing so painful, really. Because I really felt her so intensely here. And I've missed her so much this whole time."

"And did she have a message for you?"

Marilyn nods. "Yeah, it was really hard to hear. I guess I still don't want to hear it. I was expecting something else entirely."

"Because we were using an alternative therapy, you thought the exercise would tip the scales in the direction of a complementary and alternative medicine solution?"

She nods and smiles through her tears. "Something like that. My mother told me to go with what the doctors are recommending. That the tumor will kill me if I don't have the chemo, the surgery, and the radiation. She told me that if this clinical trial had been available when she was dealing with her cancer, she would still be alive right now."

"No wonder you were surprised. What do you think?"

"What can I think? This is my own mother talking to me."

I look at her sideways. "You do know, Marilyn, that this is really not your real mother, right? That you've just bridged to your own inner wisdom?"

"I believe that my mother is my own inner wisdom. They're one and the same thing to me."

I nod. "So what do you think?"

"I don't know what to think now," she replied. "I'm not as sure of myself as when I walked in here. I thought you were supposed to have all the answers."

Now it is my turn to look surprised. "Not when they keep changing all the questions."

We both smile. I can see this is about as much work as Marilyn can handle right now. Perhaps me too.

"I tell you what. For your homework assignment"—at this she mock groans—"I want you to write a letter to your mother about this whole experience. And then write one back from her to you responding to any further questions. Got it?"

"Yeah," she says, pulling on her jacket. "I got it. Too much damned homework around here."

"And bring both letters with you when you come back for the next appointment," I call after her as she leaves the room and waves a hand in the air without turning around. She's not the only one with homework to do, I think, as I consider what else may be coming down the pike.

And that's when the pager goes off.

15

THE REIKI QUEEN

It's Sylvia on 9 south. "You're still the Reiki queen around here, right?"

"Well, I won't admit to the queen title, but yes, I do Reiki."

"There's a guy up here who's just had a head and neck resection who's been asking for Reiki treatments. I didn't know who else to call."

"Sure, I can help with that. I'll be right up."

I approach Sylvia at the desk. She is charting on the computer and looks up at me.

"It's Keith Schymanski in 952. Says his ex-wife was a Reiki master so he is used to having energy work done. But the emphasis is on the ex in ex-wife so he will be grateful if you do this for him. He's still pretty raw from the surgery and is complaining more about the pain from the split-thickness skin graft on his thigh than from the operative site. You know what a bear those grafts can be."

I nod and direct myself to his room.

I always have to brace myself for the head and neck resection patients. The swelling and inflammation and skin color changes are what happens when skin is peeled away from a person's body so that the skeleton and the musculature can be worked on. The assault on these patients' body image is significant because the cutting and the resulting anatomical asymmetry is right out there in full view—not tucked behind a blouse or a pair of trousers.

Mr. Schymanski is lying on top of his sheets in a hospital gown. He is looking out the window into the grimness of the deluge, which is still pouring itself across the city, the drops pearling the windows. I knock softly on the door and enter the room.

"Mr. Schymanski, my name is Patrice. I'm the nurse Sylvia called to do your Reiki treatments. Is this a good time?"

He turns to look at me, his head and neck sutured together like something out of Dr. Frankenstein's dungeon. I keep my face composed, my eyes focused on his eyes. I want him to know that I see him in there. He plugs the trach in his throat with a finger and breathes, more than speaks, when he answers.

"Yes, please come in. I'm glad they found someone." He is a study in the effort to conserve his breath, so I indicate to him he doesn't have to talk too much. I ask him questions he can gesture about. Questions like:

"On a scale of 0-10, how bad is the pain?" He holds up eight fingers.

"Where is the pain the worst?" He points to the raw meat on his left thigh, the skin graft to which Sylvia was referring.

"I know you've had Reiki treatments before, but do you have any questions for me before I get started?"

He shakes his head no and is already closing his eyes, folding his hands together across his belly. I tell him I am going to push his bed away from the wall so I can get behind him as I begin with his head and work down. I raise the bed up to my waist level, a nod to the blown disc in my back. I unplug his telephone, so we will not be interrupted by its ring. I stand behind his bed and center my attention on the person in front of me. I rub my hands together softly, feeling the warmth of the energy flowing in a much more focused fashion, the predictable pins and needles sensation that begins to dance on the skin of my hands as I formalize a caring intention towards Mr. Keith Schymanski. And then I start.

I breathe deeply as I extend my hands to hover about an inch over his poor bloated, purpled face. Almost immediately, I feel an enormous heat wafting off him, the heat of an intense inflammation. I consciously decide that the energy I channel will be one of coolness, a blue energy that will calm down the red raw edge of the flaming heat that is surging to meet my hands. I consciously breathe in coolness, breathe out coolness, breathe in blue, breathe out blue. Consciously trying to neutralize the fiery red flames, the raw burning. I think of ice crystals, of winter stillness, of stars twinkling in a liquid, black velvet winter solstice sky.

And as I do, his breath joins in rhythm with mine.

After awhile, I move my hands to the next prescribed head position. Then the next. And the next after that. And so forth and so on until I continue over his neck. The neck with the breathing hole in it. Much like the blow hole of the great sea mammals, taking in the air and letting it go. Riding the waves of the air currents, the sea currents, the energy currents. Feeling the rhythm of his breathing in and out on the palms of my hands that hover delicately inches above his pulsating airway.

The wonder of energy work, of course, is that it is not my energy I am sending into him. So that as I channel the energy of the field we all swim in, it fills me up as he is filled. In being the conduit, my own cup runneth over. Some call it Grace, some Chi, some Prana, and still others call it by other names. All I know is that the days when I do not use it, I feel less than the days when I do. It is our birthright, our heritage. If as the physicists claim, we are all energy oscillators, flowing rivers of energy and information, why is it that the surgeon who stitched up Mr. Schymanski doesn't believe that what I am doing here is the least bit useful or helpful to him?

I watch Mr. Schymanski's face as I continue positioning my hands over his shoulders, reflecting that he will not always look like this, or feel like this, and hoping I am communicating this during the treatment. What is that coy little saying? *Nothing very, very good, or very, very bad, lasts for very, very long?* I know some folks who would take issue with that, I think.

I continue working thoughtfully down his torso, placing my hands in the prescribed positions, feeling variations in balance, flow, and temperature as I proceed. Until I get to his skin graft. The heat coming from it sears my own hands, and I once again refocus on the color blue, on using my breath to puff away little jets of chill air into the room. I spend extra time working over the skin graft.

Eventually, I finish at his feet and breathe deeply. I lower the bed back to the floor and push it to the wall again. I go to the sink to wash my hands. While I haven't touched him once, the washing helps me break the connection and clear my own field from this treatment. As I dry my hands, I look over at him resting. I am deciding I won't wake him, when I notice him looking at me, smiling. He beckons me to the bedside with a hand gesture and mouths a thank you.

I nod. "Since you're awake, can you give me a pain rating?"

He nods, holds up two fingers. "Can you come back tomorrow?" his lips form the words silently.

I smile and nod. He closes his eyes, and he's out by the time I hit the door.

GET BEHIND ME, SATAN

I run into Sylvia outside Mr. Schymanski's door and tell her he's resting comfortably and that I'll work with him again the next day.

"Gee," she says thoughtfully. "While you're here, do you mind looking in on a new patient we just received from the ED? She's an admission from the pain service, and she's in really bad shape. They are on their way up here, but if you could start working with her until they get here, it might help scrape her off the ceiling."

"Sure, that's fine," I say and she takes me to a room on the other side of the pod. The dark room is split with the bolt of the overbed fluorescent light cutting through it to the body on the bed. And the body in the bed is in such agony that it is arching its back.

"What happened?" I ask Sylvia.

"They think the catheter from her implanted pain pump dislocated out of position, so she hasn't been receiving adequate coverage. They're going to have to take her back down to the block room to reposition it. That's why she's here and why they're coming up as soon as they can. In fact, I have to go back to the

computer and see what orders came in with her from the ED."
And she's off.

I approach the patient, not even knowing her name, but I
recognize the face of suffering easily enough.

"Hi, I'm one of the nurses here. Help is on the way, but I'd
like to help you with your pain if you'll let me."

She grits her teeth, and says in a strong Appalachian accent,
"Girlie, do whatever you do, 'cause I'm hurtin real bad."

I quickly begin with a generic deep breathing exercise designed to help her relax. I introduce the notion of a light that
is moving into her body, which can softly begin penetrating
into the painful places, when she looks up at me in sheer terror.

"Get behind me, Satan!" she spits out at me fiercely. I am
absolutely taken aback. I look around me, but I'm the only
other person in the room, and she is looking directly at me.
Where is Jesus when you need him?

"I said get behind me, Satan. Don't be usin' those devilish
words with me. I know what you's tryin' to do!"

I am absolutely stunned. "I'm trying to help you relax and
breathe a little easier until the pain team arrives," I explain.

"I know evil when I see it, girlie," she hisses back at me. "I
want you outta this room right now."

And thankfully, that is when the pain team arrives, bringing with them a PCA pump and other paraphernalia that can
bring her some immediate relief before they take her downstairs.

"Glad to see you here," I say to them. "I think I upset her."

Nadine looks at me funny. "What did she say to you?" she asks as she works to get an IV needle inserted into the grimacing woman's arm.

"I think she thinks I was doing some kind of voodoo on her," I mumble apologetically.

She nods. "Mrs. MacKenzie has some real fixed notions about life. Don't you, Sara?" she asks of the woman as she opens the stopcock of the IV tubing.

"Get her outta here," the patient hisses.

"It's all right, Mrs. MacKenzie, I'm sorry I upset you. I'm leaving you in good hands."

And with that, I back out of the room and return to the nurse's station, feeling like a complete failure.

Sylvia comes back into the station and sees the expression on my face.

"What's the matter?" she asks. "Did they ever get up here?"

"Yeah, they're up here now," I say distractedly. "The patient basically threw me out of the room," I tell her, looking up at her. "I think she thought I was practicing some kind of black magic on her."

"Well, come on now, don't be too hard on yourself. It was a crisis. You didn't know her or where she was coming from. You were trying to do the best you had with what you knew at the time. You win some, you lose some. Isn't that what you're always telling us?" She looks at me kindly. I know from the neck up that she's right. But from the neck down, I feel like a failure.

"Some situations just conspire to make us feel inadequate, don't they?" she says kindly.

And I know she is right and that I will have to get over myself. The patient is in good hands; she will have her pain taken care of. I have lots of tricks in my magic bag; not all of them are everybody's cup of tea. And once again, it is a relief to know that I don't have to be all things to all people. Another little teaching coming down the pike today for my benefit, I think.

And that's when the pager goes off. Sylvia pats my shoulder and moves off to answer a ringing phone.

17

SO WHO PRAYS FOR YOU?

"Yes, it's me," I reply to the voice at the other end of the line. It's Mark down on 7 east. I'm still recovering. Time to forgive myself for not being perfect and move on.

"I know you've been working with the Broadhursts down here. Just wanted to let you know that it looks like Carl is actively dying. The family is up in the room. Didn't know if you wanted to be here for this one or not."

I so appreciate our nurses being my eyes and ears. "Thank you, Mark. I surely do. I'll be right there."

I decide to give myself a break and take the elevator down to seven. In the stall elevator is a gurney with an elderly man, the skin on his hands transparent as tissue. He has an Ommaya reservoir stitched under his scalp where he has been getting his chemotherapy infused directly into his central nervous system. He smiles at me wanly as the two transportation attendants talk back and forth over him as though he is invisible.

"I can't wait to get outta here," said one with a heavy sigh. "They've just been running me every which way today. Can't seem to catch a break."

"Mm hmm. Same here," sympathizes the other dramatically. "This is probably the worst day I've ever had here."

As the elevator door opens and I go to step out, I turn to the both of them and say, "Well, I can assure you there is someone in this elevator who is having a worse day than either of you."

I catch the old man's eye and he gives me an appreciative, if discreet, thumbs up signal, as the attendants exchange irritated glances.

Unbelievable, I think to myself. But I am already on my way to the Broadhurst room, the door of which is closed. Mark intercepts me with a freshly-brewed pot of coffee.

"How long has the vigil been going on in there?" I ask, taking the pot from him. The fragrance is intoxicating and reminds me that I was en route to get a cup for myself—how many hours ago?

"Since last night really. He is comfortable, and the place is actually jammed with friends and relatives. I may need to get more chairs in there." He pushes the door open for me as I enter, and indeed it is packed to standing room only.

In the middle of the room is the bed with a 30-something year old man in it. He wears an eye patch over his left eye, and his head has a few surgical scars tracking where his hair should have been.

His breathing is stertorous, and he is expending a lot of energy to take each breath. On the bed with him sits a large man I've seen before, a friend of Carl's, who is tenderly stroking his hand. It is a sweet sight to see such a large man be so physically affectionate with his dying friend. Carl's wife, Liz, is standing at the head of the bed, looks up, and nods me into the room. She will be left with three small children under the age of eight, but I realize they will not be left alone as I scan the room. It is filled with men and women of all ages, all sitting vigil here as Carl does his work.

"I brought you all a fresh pot of coffee," I say quietly. "Anyone need a hot refill?" A few proffer their cups gratefully and return to where they were sitting or standing. I place the pot on a bedside stand and approach Carl from the other side of the bed. I bend low to whisper in his ear that I'm here, what day it is, what time it is, and what the weather is like outside.

"And Carl, you are surrounded right now by all the people who love you. They are all here, and they all are giving you permission to do whatever the next right step is, Carl. They will all be all right."

They are all nodding in varying degrees of assent, some tearfully, some with exhaustion. But they are all nodding in agreement. I rub his shoulders gently and realize this will most likely be the last time I see Carl on this earth. I memorize his face, just one of hundreds and hundreds and hundreds, and I thank him for being such an articulate teacher, especially since his brain tumor took over.

I see that it is about time for me to leave, to give this group some privacy again. I promise someone will be looking in on them all regularly. As I turn to go, one of the women in the room who I don't know stops me.

"Is this what you do here all day?" she asks me.

"Well, some of what I do all day," I admit.

"Would it be okay if we said a prayer for you?" she asks.

I am stopped dead in my tracks. I look around the room. There must be at least 20 people in the room, and they all get up and encircle Carl's bed with me standing next to it.

"Yes, of course. I need all the prayers I can get."

And they all hold hands together, bow their heads and silently pray for me. With Carl right there, lying in the bed dying. I am so touched that the tears just stream silently down my face. Even Liz is bowing her head. Saying prayers for me.

When they all look up, I scan the circle. "I am grateful from the bottom of my heart," I tell them. "Carl is so very lucky."

The man returns to his spot on the bed and continues stroking Carl's hand. "No, we're the ones who are lucky," he says, as the group reconstitutes what amounts to its deathbed vigil tableau.

I ease out of the room and silently close the door behind me. Mark watches me approach the nurse's station and pulls out a chair for me to sink into.

"They're something else, aren't they?"

"They certainly are," I say, wiping my face with the tissue he hands me. "They certainly are." He gives my shoulder a squeeze, but just then, a doctor enters the station and asks him about a patient.

I sit there contemplating the mysteries of love and death, trying to absorb what all these people are valiantly manifesting. It overwhelms.

18

ALL HAIL TO THE CHIEF

And that's when I spot him coming down the hallway. He is a beautiful man. He has to be close to six and a half feet tall. He has a walking stick almost as tall as he is with what must be eagle feathers tied at the top. He has some sort of cowboy hat on his head with similar feathers fanned out of the front of the hatband. He is wearing a luminous cape, and I can't help noticing the boots—snakeskin or something. What do I, a city girl, know about boots? As he approaches the station, I see that he is dark with chiseled cheekbones and lustrous black hair that streams behind him as he passes. His is a commanding presence, and people in the hallway are trying not to be too obvious in their interest. But he is gorgeous. He disappears into a nearby room.

Mark turns back and smiles at me with amusement.

"Now that is something else," I say.

"Impressive, isn't he?"

I nod. "Who is he?"

"He's the son-in-law of the patient in 48 who has just been referred to hospice back on his reservation."

"Really?"

"Yeah, you should go in there. They are still finalizing the arrangements."

"But I haven't worked with that patient or the family," I respond demurely.

"No seriously, they are very open folks. I'm sure you won't regret it."

"What's going on in there right now?"

"He's ministering to her."

"Ministering? How ministering?" I ask.

"He's the chief and healer of his tribe, and he is blessing her. Really, go on in there. You'll thank me that you did."

My curiosity gets the better of me, and I quietly sneak into the room. Inside there is an elderly white woman in the bed, and a younger version of her at her bedside. The expression on the older woman's face is positively beatific. A resident and a medical student sit on the sidelines, just watching. The real person to watch is the chief. He is chanting over the woman's body. It is a haunting chant. Waving his feathered walking stick over her rhythmically. His voice is powerful, practiced, gentle. He is all concentration in this effort. His energies are poured into the woman on the bed who is a willing vessel, no doubt about it.

At a certain point, the chanting begins to slow down, and I find myself getting nervous. I am worried about the reaction of the resident and his medical student. I am worried they may not be culturally competent enough to appreciate that healing is not just relegated to conventional medicine. I am worried that I am about to have to look for a hole to crawl into.

The chanting stops. There is a profound stillness in the room.

And then the resident says, "Are you doing anything else the rest of the afternoon?"

The chief looks up at him with startling clear eyes. "No, why?"

Oh, no, I think, here it comes.

"Because I would really love it if you could make rounds with me the rest of the afternoon."

The chief smiles at him and the resident, with student in tow, reaches over to shake his hand.

"Thank you," the resident tells him. "Thank you."

I breathe a sigh of relief. Oh me of little faith!

The chief nods and watches as they exit. It is then that they notice me in the corner. I approach and introduce myself, asking if I can be of any service to them. It turns out that the white woman at the bedside is his wife, and that the woman in the bed is, as Mark said, the chief's mother-in-law. And indeed, they will be returning to the reservation, albeit with hospice care. Their needs are very simple. They are very gracious, and I find that things are well in hand. Once again today, it is I who have been ministered to.

19

THE TALE OF THE GYPSIES

I leave the room, quietly closing the door behind, as Tonya approaches me. Clearly Tonya is not happy.

"You are going to have to do something about those men in 42," she says between gritted teeth. "I am not going into that room any more. I have had it." She says it like she means it.

"Slow down," I say, and walk her to a vacant patient room nearby. "What's going on?"

Tonya is an excellent nurse, but she is also very young and unseasoned. I try to keep this in mind as I listen to her indignation. She is popping her gum faster than she can talk, hands on her hips, fairly reeking with indignation.

"It's those Gypsies!" she quips.

"Gypsies?"

"Yeah, those Gypsies in 42. Those men won't keep their cotton pickin' hands off me. I go in there to take care of her, and—I swear I am going to punch someone's lights out if they don't stop it. And I'm not the only one. They've been hassling Melinda too."

"Well, tell me what you mean by *hassling*."

"I mean I go in there to reprogram her pump or give her her meds, and they are touching my rear but pretending it's an accident."

"Are you sure? Maybe it *is* an accident." By the expression on her face, I see that it's no accident.

"Well, sounds like they have been sexually harassing you if that is the case. Do you call them on it?"

"Yes, of course, I call them on it! But they just smirk and do it again anyway. I'm telling you, I'm not going back in that room! I want a reassignment."

"Let's go talk to Jan and see what we can do about this," I say. I need more information, but it is obvious that sending Tonya back in there will do no good for anyone, least of all the patient.

We explain the problem to the charge nurse; as she listens, she begins to scan her daily assignment sheet and says she will switch Tonya with Roger to solve the problem. "I'll talk to Roger about it. We really can't have our nurses sexually harassed by that group in there."

"I can talk to them about it," I say, "but we probably should think about doing an in-service up here for the nurses on dealing with sexual harassment as it functions in the hospital. You know, as a cover for men who feel out of control, who are afraid."

"Good idea," says the charge nurse. "In the meantime, could you talk to the family about it? We need to set some boundaries, not only for the sake of the staff, but for that patient as well."

"Agreed." And with that, Tonya thanks me, and walks away with some sense of vindication. It is tough enough to be a nurse, but to be a young one in an intense environment is even tougher, regardless of where the degree came from.

As I approach room 42, I note that the name on the closed door reads Maria Romnickel. I gently knock and push the door open slowly. Which is a good thing, as I immediately hit an obstacle. The room is somewhat darkened, but I can see there are a multitude of bodies in various stages of repose on the floor on blankets and pillows. As my eyes adjust to the dim light, I see the walls are adorned with homemade religious insignia: crucifixes crudely made from masking tape and hand-written prayers. A couple of heads pop up to look at me, but soon dip back down to their pillows returning to sleep. There must be 15 people holed up in this little room, I think.

An older woman at the bedside turns to look at me and motions me inside, a finger at her lips. I gently close the door and pick my way among the sleeping bodies.

"What can I do for you?" she asks. She is a tiny bird of a woman, a woman who once must have been a great beauty. Her olive skin is lustrous; her black hair is swept back into a tight chignon at the nape of her neck. She is dressed very stylishly, her makeup is impeccable, and her gold earrings and bracelets catch what little light there is as she gestures for me to come closer so she can check me out. Her sharp eyes don't miss a thing. She gives me the once over, making no bones about it.

I introduce myself and ask how I can be of service to her and her family. She points to a younger version of herself in the bed sleeping. "My daughter," she gestures, "has the cancer in her belly. We are here to do what we can for her."

"Would you like a cup of coffee?" I ask.

She raises her eyebrows. "Yes, I think I would like that very much."

"Why don't we take it in the family waiting room, so we don't wake everyone up?"

She nods and, raising her skirt slightly, rises gracefully from the bedside as her daughter turns in her sleep. The others about the room show no sign of being disturbed. We tip-toe out, closing the door quietly as we exit.

As I settle her in an upholstered chair that seems to swallow her, I see how really tiny she is. Small, but mighty, I can't help thinking to myself. She is formidable even as she sinks back into the chair. I hand her the Styrofoam cup of steaming coffee and dive into my own even before I seat myself across from her. The warmth infuses me, and I savor the aroma as much as the flavor. I'm thankful no one else is in here, so we have some privacy.

After a moment of quiet sipping, she looks up at me with those intense, dark eyes.

"So tell me, how much do you know about us?" she asks.

"Well, this is really the first time I am meeting any of you," I say.

"No," she interrupts. "I mean about Gypsy people."

"Not a thing," I respond truthfully. "What would be important for all of us here to know?"

"Well, to begin with," she looks at me steadily. "When one of us is in trouble, we all come in from everywhere and stand together."

"Ah, that explains all the people in the room."

"Yes, we have had to work with your nurses here to permit so many of us to be in there all at once. But you see, it is our way."

I nod at this. "Is everything all right about that now?"

"Yes, but we had to promise to clear the room in case of an emergency."

"I am sure you can understand that they would need to get the emergency cart in there."

"But of course," she says, waving her hand dismissively.

"Good, I'm glad you were able to work things out to your satisfaction. It must be hard coming into our foreign little world here. Must be like being dropped on another planet."

She nods. "Well, we certainly don't live in caravans anymore, if that is what you are thinking."

"Actually, I don't know what to think. Why don't you educate me?"

"We Roma are a proud people. This particular family, while spread out all over the country, is based primarily in Chicago. You know, I live with my daughter, son-in-law, and grandchildren in their spacious house—it's 5,000 square feet—and they just put in an indoor swimming pool," she says, thumping her chest to punctuate her testimonial to the family's success. "We are in the carnival business, you see. We bring in lots of money—mostly big state fairs all across the country. We handle the concessions, the rides, the midways. We have been doing this kind of work for years. It is in our blood, you could say."

I nod as I drink my coffee, realizing how little I know of her people, how much I'll have to learn if I am to educate the staff. I sense there is a real cultural disconnect between her family and the staff. In more ways than in just the sexual harassment issue. An issue I am going to have to address, most likely here. Now.

"Tell me," I ask, "in Roma families, who is the head of the family? The matriarch or is it the patriarch?"

She smiles knowingly, shaking a finger at me. "Very good," she says. "You want to know who is the boss of the family, no? Well, if you ask the men, they will say it is them, but as you are asking me, I tell you it is me. I am the oldest female relative in this clan, but we let the men run the business. Everything else—the family—is my responsibility. Who marries who, where we live, what to do when we get sick."

"Like now? Bringing your daughter here for treatment?"

She nods as she sips. "The doctor in Chicago, when he finds Maria's tumor, he tells us to bring her here, and that your doctors will know how to fix her."

"Well, how is it going so far?"

"Oh, your treatments make her sick all the time. They tell us it is too early to know how she is doing, so we just wait with her and see."

"It must be hard for all of you to be living out of that room together. Who is taking care of the business while you are all here?"

"We are used to living together after all. We have plenty of people back home who are seeing to things until we get back."

"It is difficult nonetheless."

She nods, taking another sip, and I see her guard dropping a bit as we sip and talk together. It must be difficult to negotiate Anglo culture in a crisis. And that's what makes me think about Tonya and the staff.

"Mrs." I start to say and then realize I didn't get her name.

"Ah, call me Bella, please."

I smile and begin again, "Bella. One of our nurses came to me and is a bit uncomfortable with how the men in your family treat her when she comes in to take care of your daughter."

"Ah, I see. Your women are not used to the attentions of our men. You know, the men are—how do you say it here? Macho? They are used to giving a pretty girl the eye."

"Well if that were all they were giving them, it probably wouldn't be a problem for our nurses. I don't mean to be accusing your men, but our nurses are not used to being touched in that way, and certainly not while they are doing their work here."

She begins to make a gesture, which looks like she is dismissing the issue, so I pursue. "Bella, as the matriarch of your family, could you have a talk with the men to let them know that they are making it difficult for Maria to receive the kind of care she deserves? You don't want nurses not wanting to go into the room to take care of her, do you?"

"Of course not. But you see, my dear, they are going to get all puffed up about it. You know how the men can be."

I nod in sympathy, but she needs to understand that while they are in the hospital, they will need to abide by some of our codes of conduct just as we have tried to accommodate them.

"Think of this as trying to calm the culture wars between us. Just as the nurses have turned the other way to there being so many people in the room all at once because it is your way, can you not talk to the men about refraining from making off-color comments and touching the nurses because that is our way?"

She looks at me levelly, and I see she can find no argument in this.

"Agreed," she says finally. And on that note, an elderly woman pushing a walker opens the door and sits down across from us. She picks up one of the outdated magazines from the end table and looks at us with an air of exhaustion. "I just had to get out of that room," she says, and returns to the coverless *People* magazine.

Bella and I both look at each other and simultaneously decide that our business for the day seems to have come to a natural end.

"Can I walk you back to the room?" I ask.

She nods and says, "Only if you are going in that direction.'

"Sure." I open the door for her and ask, "Would it be all right if I look in on all of you on a daily basis while you are here? You know, to troubleshoot anything that I can help you with?"

She nods.

"And, I'd love to learn more about the Roma, too."

She breaks into a big smile, and starts picking up speed as we near the hallway where Maria's room is. As she turns the corner and heads out of sight, I notice a meeting breaking up in the conference room. Mark Howell, one of the attendings, almost hits me with the door as he rushes out.

"Oh, sorry," he quips as he downs the last bite of his sandwich.

I look past him into the room and see the table loaded with leftover sandwiches as the medical team empties around him to return to the units.

"Say, what's going to happen with all that food in there, Mark?" I ask.

He shrugs, "I don't know," and wipes his mouth with a napkin he taps into a wall receptacle. "They're all yours if you want them."

Just then, Roger turns the corner and approaches from the other hallway.

"Say Roger," I speak up to him.

"Yo," he says as he halts in front of me. Roger's an ex-corpsman.

"Hey, soldier, I understand you're taking over one of Tonya's patients."

"Yeah, I guess the boys in the room were a little too frisky for her. If they get smart with me, I'll let 'em know about it." He holds up a fist, in jest, and smiles.

"No chance of that," I say humoring him. "Say, you wanna be a hero with them right away?"

"Sure," he says, "What's up?"

"See all those sandwiches left over from the neuro rounds?"

He nods.

"Why not pass them out to Maria Romnickel's family?"

He grins, and says, "Gotcha. Wanna come with?"

"No, I think this should be your gig."

He gives me a thumbs-up sign and moves past me to gather all the sandwiches in the boxes that they came in. That should help square things away when Bella informs the boys in Maria's room to cool it, although I'm sure there will be some testing of the new rules right away. There always is. Kind of like telling a kid not to touch the wall because the paint is still wet. I'll have to get that in-service scheduled sooner than later, I think to myself.

As my mind starts to consider my schedule, a young Asian man slowly makes his way down the hall balancing himself on one side with his IV pump and on the other by a diminutive woman—most likely his wife—on the other. Every step is an effort. His capped-off nasogastric tube—pinned to the hospital gown—dangles off his taped nose. The wife looks like the paragon of devotion, and she speaks encouragingly to him in a soft dialect.

"You're doing a terrific job," I tell them as they pass by heavily. "Both of you."

They beam at me and bow slightly as they lumber on slowly, the IV wheels squeaking across the carpet. I stare after them a bit dreamily. Was that Mussorgsky's *Pictures at an Exhibition*, the ox-cart movement, rolling around in my head just then, watching their successful efforts? Just then, the pager goes off in my pocket, snapping me out of my reverie.

20

THE RED LEVER ·

"This is me," I respond into the receiver.

"Yeah, it's Roy, down here in bone marrow transplant. You've been working with the Blums, haven't you?"

"Yeah, what's up?" I reply, picturing the unfortunate young couple. Esther found out about her leukemia just about the time they returned from their honeymoon, a situation that is not as unusual as one might think. For such couples, married life is nothing short of what they might have expected to endure together after 50 years together. Unfortunately for them, they quickly become propelled into the world of premature old age: infirmity, dashed dreams, bedpans, and loss.

"She took a turn for the worse last night."

"Not again."

"Yeah, this time Saiyid says it's not reversible. They want to call it."

"That is so sad," I say mournfully. Truly mournfully. And I know that Roy is feeling that way, too. We have all adopted this young couple, and it has been hard watching her graft-versus-host disease devour her, slowly but ever so surely. The BMT unit is notorious for treating aggressively, right up to the end, especially if the patient is as young as Esther. So, if Saiyid says, this is it, then I know it must be so.

"How is David doing?"

"Well, that's why I'm calling you, actually. He's been down here all day, won't leave her side. The docs have told him that they wish this was a reversible situation, but it is definitely not. He is just standing at her bedside looking down at her. I don't think he can let her go."

The sad scene plays in my head, and I can see him watching the air from the ventilator being pushed into and out of her frail chest. In and out, in and out, in and out. And since she recovered all those previous times, why wouldn't he have the expectation that her eyelids will flutter open at the sound of his voice? God knows he's been sold on the miracles of modern high-tech medicine. And with all the hopeful residents and BMT staff reporting every single change she presents, why shouldn't he expect another miracle? Or two? Or three?

"I'm on my way," I murmur softly.

"Thanks, this is a hard one," he says sympathetically.

I hang up the receiver and sit at the desk, wondering at the why of it, knowing it is useless to ask such unfathomable questions. To know there is a large tapestry being woven and that there is nothing that is lost or wasted, does not mitigate the sadness at such suffering. And yet, my job is to help people find meaning in the suffering. To make it more bearable. Or so that line of reasoning goes.

As I rise to make my way downstairs, I pass a room where there is a transfer going on with some degree of commotion. I stick my head in the door.

"Need an extra set of hands?" I ask the nurse and the transport crew. The patient looks awfully hefty, even from here, and he looks like he is in a lot of pain.

"Thanks," the nurse says, somewhat harried. She must be new as I don't recognize her. "He wasn't supposed to be called down for his MRI for another hour and a half, but they got a quick cancellation and decided to take him earlier. I only just now gave him his pain medication for the trip, and it hasn't had a chance to kick in yet."

The patient is wincing as they start to roll him towards the stretcher. The bed is raised up as high as it can go to meet the gurney. He is red in the face and sweating profusely from the pain and the effort.

"Gosh, can we wait another 15 minutes to give the medication a chance to work?" I ask, noticing that he won't be able to help us too much in his current state.

"Nope, they said 'now.' And I guess around here, they mean it."

The patient yells out just then, and everyone stops in deference to his pain level.

"Well," I wink at the patient, who is in no winking mood. "We may not have 15 minutes, but I'm making an executive decision, and I say we have a good three."

"What good will that do?" he growls at me.

"Will you humor me?" I ask.

"That depends," he says.

"I'd like to ask you to use your imagination. Can you do that for me?"

"Look lady, just spit it out. What do you have in mind?" There's a vein in his temple that looks ready to explode from all the stress.

"Close your eyes," I reply. And he does. "Tell me, on a scale of 0 to 10, 0 being no pain, and 10 being the worst pain you can imagine, where you are on that scale right now."

"Right now, I'm at a 9," he says, the vein throbbing relentlessly.

"Okay, here's where your imagination comes in. Pretend you can see those numbers on a gauge in your mind's eye. The needle is pointing to the number nine. Can you see it?"

He is squinting, but he's nodding affirmatively. The others around the stretcher are relieved for the distraction, and making use of it to take a breather.

"Good. Now just to the right of the gauge is a red lever. Can you see the lever?"

"Yeah, I can see it," he says. One of the transporters is looking at me skeptically. I smile back at him with a finger at my lips, indicating he be patient for a few more minutes.

"Okay, I want you to put your hand on that lever, and I want you to move the lever back to a point where the reading on the gauge is going to make this transfer more bearable for you. You got it?"

"Yeah, I got it," he says.

Now the other transporter is looking at the patient with a measure of curiosity. We wait a few moments, and the nurse is looking across the bed at me with some hopefulness. Actually I am biding my time, hoping the medication begins to kick in. I am a big believer in the placebo effect. Whatever gets us where we need to be.

"Okay, where are we on the lever right now?" I ask.

"We're at a 6,"he says with surprise.

"Great, is that good enough for you?"

"Give me a few more moments. I think I can push this baby down some more," he says. The exercise has returned some measure of control to him, and he is responding to that dynamic. Taking charge.

The one transporter leans over to me gingerly, and whispers "He's into it," and shrugs in amazement.

"I think that's as far back as I can get it," he says, and he visibly relaxes his internal efforts.

"Well, where are we now?" I ask.

"We're just under 5," he says and opens his eyes.

"Why your eyes are very blue," I say, smiling down at him. "Didn't notice it before when your face was so red."

He grins, and is actually able to help us scoot him over a bit onto the stretcher. As the transporters raise the sidebars, the nurse says, "Well, I learn something new every day."

"You and me both," I quip back at her, and the transporters sail out of the room.

21

REQUIEM FOR THE HONEYMOONERS

I suddenly remember that I need to get down to BMT and swing around to take the elevators. As I swipe my ID card to gain access into BMT, I notice Roy hanging up the phone at the station. Saiyid, one of the attendings on the unit, is writing orders beside him. His trim moustache and goatee give him an air of distinction, his dark eyes an air of knowing.

"Roy told me you were coming down to see the Blums," Saiyid says. "I'm glad you're involved. He doesn't seem to hear that she is not going to make it this time."

"I will promise to do all I can," I say, but then decide to go further, looking him in the eyes, "if you will ask your staff to stop reporting to him any kind of miniscule changes no matter how positive. It doesn't matter if you've told him that her blood chemistries are down the tubes if you tell him that her creatinine has improved by .000000005%, because that is all he is going to hear."

"I know, I know. Our staff is having trouble being the bearers of bad news," Saiyid says. "I will tell them."

We look at each other levelly. "This is hard for all of us."

"Thanks for coming down and working with them."

As he turns to go, I say, "Saiyid, I appreciate everything you've been trying to do for them. Remember, death is not the enemy here."

"Well, if it isn't, then I don't know what is," he says glumly as he continues down the corridor.

"The poor docs and their wizard complexes," Roy says, shaking his head looking after him. He looks back at me and says, "David's still in the room."

"And I'm still on my way," I say as I head down the hall. I peer into the isolation room and see David white-knuckling the bedrail as he hovers over Esther. I push the door in just a little.

"Would you like some company?" I ask David.

He turns to see who has disturbed the solitude. His face is worn. He looks much older than his 26 years. I can tell from his clothes that he probably slept in them, likely in the family waiting room. His flannel shirt is wrinkled, and he still has "bed head."

"Sure, come on in, if you like," and he returns his gaze to the body lying in front of him.

I go to the anteroom sink where I scrub up. I cannot imagine being David. I cannot imagine what I am about to say to him. I just cannot imagine.

I gently push the door back open, and he makes room for me at her bedside. Esther, who used to be this vivacious redhead, is now so pasty that she blends into her bed sheets. Her little body looks shrunken, wizened. There is a touch of blue to her lips, to her nail beds. Her little chest is being pumped up and down. Relentlessly.

"David, I just can't imagine what you must be thinking here as you look at Esther."

"No, I don't suppose you can." I hear a touch of anger. Just a touch.

"It must be hard to believe that after all the work the two of you have put into this that you find yourselves here. Now." For some reason, the Beuters from earlier in the day pop into my head. Déjà vu all over again.

He says nothing. Just keeps examining her face. Her poor little face haloed by the tarnished peach fuzz ringing her scalp.

"Are you here alone?"

He slowly shakes his head. "No, Jerry and Rose are down in the cafeteria for a cup of coffee," he says, referring to Esther's parents.

"I'm glad you're not here by yourself. It is too much for any one person to have to handle alone," I say quietly.

He turns his red-rimmed eyes towards me. "But you see, I am alone. I am supposed to know what to do here. And I don't." He is exhausted, consumed by an event that spun out of control months and months ago. He spins the wedding ring on his finger.

"I can't believe it has all come to this," he says finally.

There is really nothing to say to this. I place my hand softly on his hand and he lets me. We stand that way for some time watching Esther's face. I think of the children this couple will never have, the trips never taken, the holidays never celebrated. There really is no justice in this world, I think.

"And so, David," I say softly, gently. "If Esther were standing here right beside us. Right now. Looking down at the body lying here on this bed. What would she say she would want?"

He removes his hand from mine and squeezes his fingers against his eyes. "I knew you were going to ask me that question," he says tersely.

I wait him out. I know he is angry. I wait him out.

The arm drops limply and he slumps forward, resting his forearms on the bedrails.

"I know she wouldn't want this," he says. "This is not life. And it's not death either. It's a living death."

"What do Jerry and Rose say?"

"They are hurting so much they can barely speak. They used to cheerlead us ad nauseum. But you know, I don't think even they have it in them to cheerlead us any more."

"What makes you say that?"

"They told me they would back whatever decision I made. But I wish I was in the position to say that to them. I don't want to be stuck with the responsibility of this."

"So Esther never told any of you what she would want if it came to this?"

"Nope—part of the cheerleading pact. You know: 'be positive.'"

"Ah yes, the prison of positive thinking."

He nods.

Just then, there is a mild rap at the door. Jerry and Rose, returning from the cafeteria.

Rose smiles at me and says, "Any changes?"

I look in David's direction, steering her there nonverbally.

"Nope. The same," he says, never removing his eyes from Esther's face.

Jerry nods his head at me as they join our little circle around the bed.

"I know it must seem incredible to you that Esther is not rallying, like she has in the past," I say, clearing my throat.

Rose starts to cry. I can see she is exhausted. Jerry puts his arm around her as she sways at the bedside, her hand at her throat.

"The most unnatural thing," she chokes out. "You can't imagine . . . to watch your child die."

David looks up at her. I see it is the first time she is acknowledging the reality of the situation in front of him. She has used the "D" word.

"You know there is no ethical difference between withdrawing life support and not having started it in the first place if the treatment is considered futile. There is no major religion in the world today that would disagree with that. You also know it is a lot to ask of one person to make the decision to withdraw life support at a time like this."

They all nod.

No responses from anyone. Just the thump and swish of the ventilator as the air is pumped into and out of that tiny little chest.

Rose takes hold of Esther's limp hand and caresses her bald head. "My sweet girl," she murmurs. She looks up at David.

"You have been a good husband to my daughter, David. Jerry and I appreciate what you gave her these many months. You made her life more bearable because you were in it."

I am noticing all the past tense phrasing she is using. I am sure David is noticing it, too. Moments go by. No one says anything.

"And so, Rose," I say. "If Esther were standing here with us looking down at this body, what would she say she would want for herself?"

Rose looks up at me with the eyes of a Pietà. "Not this," she finally says. She looks at Jerry who looks back at her in anguish, and he nods. They both look at David.

"David?"

"Not this," he mouths in agreement. We all stand in silent tribute as we understand that over the many months, tiny shifts have taken place beneath the surface. Little shifts that never registered at the surface, but yet registered beneath it nonetheless. And here, now, suddenly an earthquake of a decision that seems to have come out of nowhere. Yet really it hasn't. Because the tiny shifting has been pulling the fault lines apart all along. A threshold has been crossed. Here. Now. There is a palpable sag in everyone's shoulders. A sense of surrender. I give it a moment, and then I say, "What you

are doing here is such a high call to love. How lucky Esther is
to be surrounded by people who love her so dearly."

Tears all around. Including me. "May I?" I ask David as I
reposition myself at Esther's ear. He nods, wiping his nose.

"Esther, you are surrounded by people who love you, David, your mother and your father, all of whom are sending
their love to you to do with it whatever is your next right
step. Everyone in this room is sad, but everyone in this room
will be okay with whatever it is you decide you need to do
next. They will make it possible for it to be your decision,
Esther." I realize, not for the first time today, that I am giving
this little speech. I wonder how many more times are ahead
of me yet today, and just as suddenly, don't want to know.

I rise up slowly, giving her a little peck on the cheek. Jerry,
Rose, and David can't see for tears, and I realize it is time for
me to give them some privacy. I silently squeeze David's arm
and back out of that room, where something momentous,
something sacred, is transpiring. As I walk out of the unit,
I wonder how long it will take before they withdraw all the
bells and whistles and let nature take her rightful course. I
pray for all of them. And as usual, I am humbled by what I
see in them.

Some states have shifted to AND, Allow Natural Death,
instead of DNR, Do Not Resuscitate. The former sounds
more natural, the latter sounds harsh, withholding. Breathing machine. What family is going to remove a breathing
machine from their loved one? The more accurate description
is a mechanical ventilation machine. Because what Esther is
doing in there is not really breathing. Feeding tube. What

family member is going to remove a feeding tube? The more accurate description is chemical sustenance. What Esther is doing in that room is not eating.

Language is very important.

I stop in the staff restroom to wash my face. I look into the mirror and realize I look so very tired. I wonder if I've been walking around looking like this. I look like death warmed over, but I feel very much alive.

Very much alive.

The restroom door closes behind me and I dawdle in the corridor, trying to get a hold of myself. Again.

And that's when the pager goes off.

22

WEDDING BELLS

"Yes?"

"Hi, it's Jamie up on 10. Wanna hear something fun."

"I could use some fun news. Whatcha got?" I ask, trying a bit unsuccessfully to enter into the mood of the moment.

"We're going to have a wedding up here!"

I know this is supposed to be fun. But we all know that really good news about weddings would mean the couple is holding the wedding *outside* of the hospital, not in it. Weddings here usually mean that someone is making memories, a commitment. Not necessarily a commitment that will last a long time.

Still, and even so, a wedding is a celebration of life, love, of relationship. A wedding is a profession of faith and hope. And as such, it is good news and deserves to be celebrated.

"Let me guess," I query. "You want me to round up some flowers from the fifth floor, right?"

"You got it," she says." Do you have time?"

"For you? Of course I have time. Where is the betrothal to take place?"

"In room 1045 in an hour."

"Do you want me to call Pastoral Care?" I ask, trying to think ahead.

"They're already in the loop."

"Always a pleasure to work with you, Jamie. I'm on my way."

"See you soon," she says.

Grateful for the break in the litany of the day's many sadnesses, I swing up to the executive suite, nabbing a cart with wobbly wheels on the way. As the elevator opens into the main corridor, I spot a beautiful bouquet of silk lilies in shades of pearly pastels—peaches and creams—with feathery palm fronds. I swipe it from the credenza, peek into the executive conference room, and see no one inside. I open the door, swinging the cart into the room smartly and begin to clear the shelves of silk ivy, birds of paradise, and peonies that are a riot of improbable hues. I am wondering how I can make off with the fake fig tree in the corner when the CEO happens into the room.

"Don't tell me," he groans with fake pleasure, "Another wedding."

"Yup, you wanna come, Ted?"

"I would love to, but I'm on my way to a meeting with Jeff." He gives me a closer look. "Say, are you okay? You look a little ragged around the edges."

"I'm fine. Thanks for asking."

"It looks like you've been crying. Having trouble coping today?" His bemused grin is a concerned one, nonetheless.

"Yes, I have been crying, and yes, that is coping here."

He comes up to help me nab a silk hydrangea arrangement off the top shelf, and as he puts it on the cart, he gives me a brief hug.

"Thanks for all you do here," he says with a crooked grin. And then as he leaves for his meeting, follows with "and see that you keep it up."

I appreciate our little family here, looking out for one another. I really do.

Once the cart is covered with enough silk blooms to blanket the hospital, I wheel it back to the elevators. The doors open, and I am met with the dazzled expressions of what appear to be some happy home-goers. The middle-aged woman in the wheel-chair admires the spray of flora.

"Well, someone's going to feel lucky today." She is beaming, and the man who is wheeling her down to the ground floor is looking equally beamy.

"You have no idea," I reply. "Blowing this popcorn stand, are we?"

"You bet," she says. "I am so grateful to all of you here. I am leaving this place cancer-free. Hope I don't ever have to darken your doors again."

"Well, then, not to seem too unfriendly, but I guess I hope I never see you again," I concur, sharing in their celebratory relief.

"No offense taken," the handsome gentleman says. "We feel truly blessed."

The door opens and they make their way off the elevator amidst a jumble of plastic hospital bags stuffed with various personal items. I watch them roll towards the exit and realize that I don't come into contact enough with the people who receive good news here. Of course, the nature of my work keeps me amongst those who are delivered the bad news.

The doors close again, and I push my floor button, lost in my own thoughts, although I can't say what they are. When the doors open, I am pointed down the hallway to the hospital room that's being transformed into a bridal bower. There is a young man lying in the bed. He is extremely thin, which gives his large eyes the specter of a luminescent being from another planet. Distinctly other-worldly.

"Well come in, come in," he says, grinning. "I take it you are here to transform my cave into something more resembling a chapel?"

"Indeed I am, sir," I say entering into the conviviality of the moment. "And do I take it that you are the lucky groom?"

"You may, you may," he says waving me in. "I'm Jack. Thanks for helping us out here. These are great," he points to the flowers.

"Congratulations, Jack. I'm Patrice. Is there any special way you want me to decorate your boudoir here?"

"Naw," he says, "I'll leave it up to your judgment."

"Great. Well, I'll get started then," and I move hospital supplies and equipment into closets, the bathroom, and behind doors. As I begin spreading around the greenery, a couple of young men enter the room carrying what looks to be a tuxedo bag.

"Whoa, what do you guys think you're up to?" laughs Jack, eyeballing the suit. I can see he's surprised, but also pleased and excited. Almost a little feverish, if I didn't know any better.

"You don't think we could let you get hitched looking like a derelict do you?" one of them shoots back, hanging up the bag on a door hanger.

"Meet my brothers," Jack says as he introduces us.

"I can certainly see the family resemblance," I say. "What a great idea," I nod to the bag as one of them helps me take a particularly large vase of mixed posies off the cart. The other brother takes the tuxedo out of the bag and I can see it is just the top part—a shirt, jacket, tie, and cumberbund. This will definitely be a bedside service.

"When does the bride get here?" I ask.

"Probably in half an hour or so," Jack says as one of his brothers begins to help him out of the patient gown. "Hope you can come back here and join us. It will be the event of the season, I can assure you." He is grinning to beat the band.

"Thanks for the invite, Jack. I'm going to give you boys some privacy as you prepare for your bride."

"Great," he says as he is lost in a gaggle of arms and elbows as they try to get him into the monkey suit, difficult enough to get into when able bodied and not bed-bound with a central line pouring out of your chest. I close the door behind me, not being able to wipe the grin off my own face. Jamie passes me by in a hurry on her way into another room, blond hair flying behind her.

"Is he cute or what," she flings behind her. It isn't a question.

23

OCCUPATIONAL HAZARDS

As I lean against the closed door, I happen to catch a glimpse of Beth who must have just stepped off the elevator. About the same time, she spots me and motions me to follow her. Beth is the nursing operations officer for the hospital. It is her job to administer the day to day running of the units, to make sure everybody has everything they need to get the job done. It is also her job to deal with the crises that are a predictable part of every hospital day.

I catch up with her. She hasn't slowed down at all.

"Where's the fire?" I ask, a bit out of breath. I'm short and can't keep up with her long stride.

"So far, no fire today," she says, and I know she isn't kidding. "But I did just get a call. Sheryl Snell just stuck herself with a needle." She looks at me pointedly. "The patient is HIV positive."

"Oh my God," I say, and propel myself forward to keep up with her. "How's she doing?"

"Chris says she's having a meltdown."

"Well, just because she gets a needle stick doesn't necessarily mean . . ."

"I'm already ahead of you," Beth interrupts. "You know that, and I know that, but I don't think Sheryl's having any of it. Infection Control and Employee Health have just been called and they're already onboard. They should be here any moment now."

Nurses, needle sticks, and back injuries. Like fish to water, like Mom and apple pie, like French fries and cheeseburgers. Nurses and needle sticks.

We round the corner and knock softly on the nurse manager's office door. Carla Honan's voice asks who is there.

"It's Beth and Patrice," Beth says.

"Come on in," the voice responds.

We enter the office. Carla is kneeling by the chair where Sheryl's tear-stained face pops up at us. She is definitely having that meltdown, and we close the door behind us.

"Can you believe I did this?" she says. "23 years as a nurse. Can you believe I did this?"

Beth looks at Carla, and Carla just shakes her head imperceptibly. I put my hand on Sheryl's shoulder.

"Sheryl, don't go jumping to any conclusions about this now."

She looks at me. "Don't try to cheer me up," she says with a scowl. "It's not going to work."

I nod, knowing that most likely I would be scared too if this happened to me. There is another knock at the door.

"Who is it?" Carla asks. She is trying to protect Sheryl's privacy in all of this. What a good soul!

"It's Emile from Infection Control," the voice returns.

Since I'm by the door, I open it, and Emile steps in the room. Before he can get it closed, Jane Woodruff from Employee Health slips in behind him. She's carrying a phlebotomy tray.

"Thanks for coming," Beth says. "She's thinking the worst, Emile."

I move out of the way as Emile stoops down to be at eye-level with Sheryl.

"I know you are scared to death right now," he says earnestly. "But not everyone who is stuck with an HIV needle, gets HIV, okay? In fact, the chances are pretty remote."

"Easy for you to say," Sheryl whimpers. "I just cannot get over the fact that I did this."

"It was an accident, Sheryl," Beth says calmly. "We all have them."

"Not like this," Sheryl returns dryly.

Jane gestures to Emile that she would like to get in closer to Sheryl to take a blood sample. He makes room for her. Suddenly it feels like we are all ganging up on Sheryl. I move away.

"Sheryl, I'm going to be quick," she says as she ties the tourniquet off and starts patting the inside of Sheryl's elbow raising a vein.

"Well, don't be too quick," Sheryl whimpers, "or someone will have to get a blood sample from you too."

The two look at each other as Jane slaps on a pair of gloves and makes quick work of the stick.

"How long will it take to confirm this one way or another?" Beth asks Emile.

"Should have the results back in one to two weeks."

"That long? How am I going to be able to function for one to two weeks?" Sheryl cries.

Carla says, "Sheryl, I'm going to have someone drive you home today. You're in no shape to work. I see you have the next two days off anyway. I'll call you tomorrow and see how you're doing. We can talk more about a plan then." She looks in Beth's direction, and Beth nods in agreement.

Jane gets off the floor with her sample, and she and Emile head for the door. Emile looks back at Sheryl. "Sheryl, I can't stress enough how minimal the risk is from this one exposure."

"Really?" she asks.

"Really," he says. "You're not alone in this. I'll be staying in touch with you, okay?"

Sheryl looks down at the floor and nods, "Okay."

They leave and Carla picks up the phone. "I'd like to call James. I think it would be a good idea for him to pick you up and take you home."

Sheryl nods and gives her James' work number. Carla briefly tells him what's happened, what the plan is. "Thanks, James, I'll tell her. Bye." She looks at Sheryl. "What a guy. He's leaving work right now to come and pick you up."

Sheryl smiles through her tears. "He's a good man," she says. She looks around the room. "Thanks, you guys, for being here. I'm a mess."

Beth squeezes her shoulder. "Wouldn't be anywhere else."

Sheryl smiles at that. "I'm okay," she says. "I'll just wait for James here. I'll be okay, really." I think she's reassuring herself more than she is reassuring the rest of us.

Carla looks at me and Beth. "Yeah, thanks for coming over so fast. Everything happened so quickly."

We both nod, and I make a mental note to call her tomorrow to follow up on Sheryl's status. It's going to be a long week or two. Waiting has always been my own personal agony. I don't envy her that.

We edge out of the room, closing the door behind us.

"What do you think?" I ask Beth.

"I'm going to think positive unless I hear differently," Beth shrugs. "Hey, thanks for coming with me. I'll see ya around the neighborhood." She gives me a wan grin and disappears around the corner, on to the next fire she needs to put out.

And that's when the pager goes off.

24

PREGNANT WITH TROUBLE

"Yes?"

It's Roberta from one of the outpatient clinics. "Can you come down to the second floor. Chris Satullo just met with a young gal who is two months pregnant. She's just diagnosed her with a breast cancer and has told her that she doesn't think it's a good idea for her to postpone her treatment until after her delivery. The patient is very upset."

"What a nightmare," I say, but this hasn't been the first time for such a scenario, and it won't be the last. "I'm on my way."

As I approach the appointment desk, I see Chris Satullo handing a pile of charts to the receptionist. She turns to me and says, "Roberta fill you in?"

"Not with the details," I say as she leads me back into her consultation office. Chris has a wonderful mix of technical and interpersonal skills, which makes her a favorite physician with patients and nurses. If I had to go through this, I would want to go through it with Chris.

"Jennifer Chubb is 27 years old and is eight weeks pregnant. She's got a fairly large tumor, and we need to start treatment immediately. If she were maybe seven or eight months pregnant, I'd be more willing to wait. I really think at this point, it is really too dangerous to put off her treatment for half a year, waiting for her to deliver. A real issue here is the fact that she is Catholic, and the abortion thing is really taboo."

"Yes, but the church does not expect her to carry a child to term if it will endanger the life of the mother."

"Right, but she is having trouble hearing that from me," Chris says. "I've spent as much time with her as I possibly can, but you can see what's out here," she says waving at the waiting room full of more souls in various states of chemo servitude. "I'd appreciate it if you could do some intensive work with her. Really, time is of the essence here. Let me know what happens when you are done, okay?" she says as she knocks softly on a nearby door and takes the chart off the hanging rack. She pastes a smile on her face and greets her next patient. "Hey, Mr. Chen, how are you?" I hear her say as the door closes behind her.

I see Roberta out of the corner of my eye, and she points me to the exam room where Jennifer awaits me. I stop momentarily outside the room, listening, but hear no sounds from within. I knock softly on the door, and think I hear someone mumbling something on the other side, but it is difficult to make out whether I am bid entrée or not. I softly push open the door. Inside is a young man and a young woman, both of them with red-rimmed eyes, both of them looking up at me, both of them looking like they have been through wars. She has close-cropped black hair, and is twisting a wad of tissues over and over in her hands. He is tall, muscular, protective seeming and keeps his eyes locked on her worn face. The energy in the room is one of desperation.

"Hi, I'm Patrice, one of the nurses here. Did Dr. Satullo tell you to expect me?"

He nods, stands, and shakes my hand, "Yes, she did. I'm Steven Chubb, and this is my wife, Jennifer." Numbly, he backs down into his chair beside his wife.

Jennifer looks up briefly, nods, and continues to worry the tissues. I offer her some clean ones, and she tosses the old ones away.

"Dr. Satullo has shared with me what you are facing. It must be impossible to absorb all this."

Steven waits for Jennifer to speak. When she doesn't, he turns to me politely. "Well, yeah, it is impossible to even consider what she is suggesting. Jen and I have been trying to have a baby for the last two years. And now that she's pregnant, this doesn't seem fair. Or right."

I look toward Jennifer who stares blankly at the floor.

"Jennifer, what are you thinking?"

She takes a moment. I can see she is still in a state of shock, that much of this conversation may not even be remembered later and will most likely have to be repeated.

"Well, it's like Steven says. I can't imagine giving her up," she rubs her belly. It still looks flat.

"You know it's a girl?"

"More like I feel it's a girl," she says smiling wanly.

I nod. She has already begun to imagine this soul into being. I remember fantasizing like this when I was pregnant myself. My heart aches for her.

"Which is why I can't give her up," she says looking dead-on at me. "I don't think that God would have given her to us if he thought we couldn't take care of her. We are in God's hands. I am putting my faith in God."

"Sounds like your faith is very important to you."

"We're Catholic," she nods, as if that is all the explanation needed.

"So your religious values are informing this decision."

She nods.

"Did Dr. Satullo make it clear what would happen to you if you should wait the half year or so before starting treatment?"

"Yes, she did. But it's a chance I'm willing to take," she replies. "I can carry her to seven months, have a C-section, and get started on my treatment then."

"What if that's too late?"

"What if it isn't?"

"That is always a possibility. None of us here has a crystal ball. However the doctor is worried that will put you at unreasonable risk considering the staging of your tumor, and the probability that it has already metastasized."

"I understand that, but I truly believe that all things are possible with God."

"So you might live to deliver your baby, but you might orphan her by doing so," I put gently.

She looks at me levelly. "As you say, none of us has a crystal ball."

Well, I can see we are going to go round and round here. I know when I am outgunned, so I decide to call in the big guns.

"Since your faith is so important to you, I wonder if it would be helpful to talk to a priest about this."

They look at each other, and Steven turns to me. "We have our priest back in our home parish, but I'm not sure how much experience he has dealing with this kind of situation."

I nod. "Well, our Catholic chaplain here has lots of experience with this situation. If he has time now, do you have time to talk to him about it?"

They look at each other, and she shrugs her assent.

"Sure," Steven says. "We took the whole day off for this appointment. We can stay to talk with him."

"Let me see if I can arrange it. I'll be right back," and I get up, turn as I close the door behind myself. Jennifer is twisting the tissues, and Steven is rubbing her shoulder protectively. Too young to have to figure this out, I think. But as the saying goes, life comes at you fast, and often we learn by flying by the seat of our pants. On the job training, I think.

I find a phone at the reception desk.

"Hi, Greg. Am I interrupting something?"

"No," he says, "just on my way into a room to administer the last host of the day. What's up?"

Greg's realization of his role as a priest ministering to the sick is fairly close to ideal. None of the pat, cliché answers for questions that don't have any. No preaching. No dogmatics. He is just a font of compassion. I explain the situation to him. He listens thoughtfully. Responds quickly.

"Listen, let me just go ahead and give communion here, and I'll be right down, okay?"

"Thanks, Greg." I return to the room where they remain, just as when I left them.

"Father Greg will be down in a moment," I say. "I explained the situation you are up against."

"Tell me. What would you do if you were me?" the young woman asks, narrowing her eyes.

I look at her squarely. "I've gotten to the point in my life where I know that unless I am actually in the situation, I have no idea what I'd do until I get there."

She nods. "Do you have children?"

"Yes," I say. "One son."

"I think people who already have children may forget what it's like to want them and not have them."

"I don't envy you this decision."

Just then, there's a quiet knock at the door.

"Come in," I say, and Greg walks through the door. He is a young man in full collar. I am so appreciative that he could respond so quickly. We tend to watch each other's backs and roll up our sleeves for each other when asked. When it comes to dealing with such issues, it is definitely a team effort. I make introductions. He listens carefully to Jennifer as she explains her thinking.

"Of course, you do know that Mother Church does not believe that in this situation, the life of the child supersedes the life of the mother," he comments gently.

"I understand, Father. But I just don't know if I would be able to live with myself afterwards, you know? How do I forgive myself for being so imperfect in this respect?"

So that's it. Imperfect. She can't forgive herself for the situation she is in. She is feeling responsible for creating her own dilemma, perhaps for creating her own cancer.

Greg picks up on this as well. "What is it that you need to be forgiven for, Jennifer?" His face is so imploring, so non-judgmental, so filled with kindness. I see her watching his face carefully and understand that for her, Greg is the face of God in the room. I know Greg understands this, as well. It is a rather large burden to be carrying. And yet he does so with Grace.

She looks at Steven, her face in a grimace. "Steven, I am so sorry. Steven, I am so sorry." She weeps.

Steven is looking at her in surprise and wraps his arms around her. My heart goes out to Steven. He knows that one way or another he is going to lose someone here—be it the baby or Jennifer. But he is going to lose someone nonetheless.

"Hey, babe, nothing to forgive here. Nothing to forgive." He rocks her.

"I am so sorry. I have let you down, let me down, let this baby down." She weeps. They rock.

Greg brings his chair in a little closer to them. "Jennifer, God is sending this situation to you for a purpose. What is it that you have to learn from this situation that it has been created for you?"

She looks up at him. "I have no idea," she says. "Why would God do such a thing?"

He looks her steadily in the eye. "Promise me, Jennifer, that you will not make a permanent decision about this until you can answer that question." He takes her hands in his own. "Promise me."

She looks into his face. And then she slowly nods. He takes out a card from his pocket and hands it to her. "I think this is way too big of a decision to be making right now. I would very much like it if you could sleep on it overnight. And perhaps, we could set up another time to meet in the next couple of days. Certainly it is important enough to merit that kind of time, don't you think?" He nods his head, eyes locked with hers, and she shortly entrains her head nodding to his.

She looks over to Steven who says, "Sounds reasonable to me, babe."

"Okay, I guess we can do that," she says. "But I think I've already made up my mind on this," she warns him.

"Let's just let it rest for now, and we'll see where we are in a couple of days when you've had a chance to digest all this. Meanwhile, I have a pamphlet I'd like you to read before we get together again. It might help you one way or another." He pulls a pamphlet from his pocket and hands it to her.

"In the meantime, I'm praying that your decision is in the highest good of all concerned. Would you like a moment of prayer now?" And that simple question serves to reaffirm his position as the church's emissary.

She and Steven both nod and bow their heads. I bow mine as well.

"Lord, grant us the wisdom and compassion to know what is being asked of us, to use the gifts we've been given so that our hands become Your hands in this world. Lord, help us remember to keep each other, to cherish one another, and to hold ourselves larger than we thought capable of. Amen."

"Amen," we all say, looking up at one another. The prayer clears the air, puts us all on the same team, centers our caring intentions. The prayer was definitely the way to go.

We rise and shake hands with each other, agreeing to reconvene in a few days. We watch them leave, Steven helping Jennifer on with her coat. We watch them make their way down the corridor to the lobby.

"Well, Greg, what do you think?"

He watches them. "I think it can go either way," he says. "I guess we wait and see." He gives my arm a friendly squeeze and follows the couple down the hall.

And that's when the pager goes off.

25

TROUBLE IN PARADISE

"It's Bronson Thibadoux," Murphy's voice growls on the line.

"Let me guess," I smile, shaking my head ruefully. "He bought you all pizzas the first night he came in, and now he is driving you all crazy."

"You got it," Murphy replies. "If you don't do something with him, we are all going to kill him."

"Now I know that you know it's the steroid burst that's doing this to him," I begin.

"You know it, we know it, and Bronson knows it, but we're going to kill him anyway."

"I'll take a turn with him," I say. Poor Bronson. Poor everyone. Bronson's monthly chemotherapy for six months includes a round of industrial-strength steroids to mitigate side effects. Unfortunately for Bronson, and for everyone around him, the steroids transform him from an exuberant and quirky personality into an over-bearing bully. And it doesn't take long. Usually, the first night he comes in, he has a party for the staff, usually with carry-out brought in. Bronson likes to party. Everybody is one big happy family.

By day three, he has terrorized everybody on staff, offered to sue anybody who darkens his door, can't find a kind thing to say to anybody, and has basically exhausted everyone to the point of annihilating him. Then he is discharged. The steroids are weaned down to nothing, and he becomes a playful kitten again. Until the next round when it starts all over again, and Bronson returns, feeling embarrassed and sheepish about his previous stay, and tries to make it up to everybody. When you are with him 24/7 for a week, the way his nurses are, it is easy to forget that it is the steroids you are dealing with, not Bronson. This is only month number three. There are three more rounds to go after this.

I rap on the door softly, and Bronson's voice commands, "Enter." I peek in the door. He gives me the eye, waves me in, and continues with his phone call.

"I told you, Jimmie, I don't like that shade of red. You tell those guys to repaint the entire room, or I am not paying for the job! I know I picked that color, but it didn't turn out to match the chip. Listen, Jimmie, I am the customer, and I am always right. I don't care how they do it, just tell them to do it, or I'm not paying."

He returns the phone to its cradle and turns towards me, his satin red pajamas a stark contrast against the utilitarian hospital bed linens.

"Trouble in Paradise, Bronson?" I ask, taking a seat by the bed.

"Very funny," he says. His revue club, which he is renovating, is indeed called "The Paradise." "What are you doing here?"

"Thought I'd come by and see how you're doing."

"I bet they sent you in here, didn't they," he jerks his head toward the door. He's all rumpled feathers.

"Bronson, are you feeling like it's 'them against you?'"

"Don't start that psychobabble with me," he sneers.

"I just want you to remember that this is the steroids talking, and not you."

"Why don't you remind them of that," he retorts.

"Okay, I will, if you'll remember it too, and settle down here a bit. I feel like I walked in here with a bull's eye painted on my chest."

"Just remember that this is what you guys are doing to me. I didn't ask for it."

"I understand," I say it at least to placate him a little so we can move on from square one. It helps that I am once removed from his direct care, that I am not the one sticking him, giving him his drugs, or even ordering them. It makes me appear more neutral, and I try to take advantage of that.

He continues to fuss and fume, looking for something he can't find on his over-the-bed table. "Damn attendant can't clean up this mess," he grumbles. He finally finds what he's hunting for. It's a hand mirror. He looks into it and rolls his eyes.

"Marco thinks I should just get this head buzzed."

"What do you think?"

"I think I'm tired of looking like a freakin' cancer patient." And he slams the mirror down on the bed.

"So what's this really about, Bronson?"

He gives me a long and steady glare that eventually softens since I don't back down.

"What if I'm going through all this, and it still doesn't work?"

"Okay, so what if that does happen?" I ask.

"Well, then, what am I doing all this for?" he yells back at me. "Look at me. I'm a circus freak!"

"I know your appearance is very important to you, Bronson," I return softly.

He again looks at me and throws up his hands in exasperation. I take a chance and move in closer.

"You know, Bronson, I'm not going to just pat you on the hand and tell you everything is going to be all right. Because I just don't know that. I will tell you that I remember that you signed up for this because we all thought—including you—that it was the best chance you had of beating this thing. We all still do. And until that proves not to be the case, I'm going to believe it until you can believe it for yourself."

He meets my gaze, and then turns to look out the window.

"You know, Marco is much younger than me. I'm worried that he's not going to stick around for all the bells and whistles. He didn't know he was signing up for this when we hooked up." He picks at his nails. "I look old. I look like hell."

"Have you talked with him about this?"

He shakes his head, again not meeting my gaze. "No, I'm afraid to."

"Afraid to hear that he's thinking about leaving?"

"That. And afraid to hear that he might not." He edges himself out of bed and pushes his IV pole over to the bathroom. I wait for him to finish as he edges over to the sink to wash up.

"You're feeling vulnerable having Marco watch you go through this," I hazard to guess.

"Vulnerable? Exposed is more like it," he sneers as he ambles back into the bed. He throws a burgundy chenille wrap around his shoulders.

"I love that color," I tease him to give us both a chance to lighten up. He throws me a mock dirty look as he eases back into pillows cased in satin brocades of maroon, claret, crimson, scarlet, and ruby. Hardly hospital issue.

"You know, Bronson, it's not uncommon for partners to be going through serious illness with each other."

"If you're referring to the 'other epidemic,' at least that has a political correctness about it that I could at least wear as a badge of courage."

"I cannot believe you even said that," I say, somewhat appalled in spite of myself.

He looks at me ruefully. "I guess I should be talking to Marco."

I nod. "If you don't, I think the staff will commit suicide or homicide. And I'd be placing bets on the latter."

He grins at me sheepishly. "Tell them I'm sorry. I'll try to do better."

I get up and give him a hug. "Tell them yourself, you big lug."

He nods. The phone rings, and he answers it as I leave the room. As the door closes, I hear him yelling into the receiver, "I told you that it's not dark enough, you idiot. I'm warning you, I'm not going to pay for it if I'm unhappy."

26

WORLDS COLLIDE

As I turn the corner and head into the other pod, I hear a high-pitched wailing. It is compelling, coming from one of the corner rooms. Patients and family members are coming to their doorways to see what is going on. As I approach the room, Lorna intercepts me.

"What's going on?" I ask.

"It's Mr. McPherson. He's just died. That's his wife in there. Can you see if you can get her to quiet down? She's freaking out the other patients up here. I've tried to talk to her about it, but I don't think she understands me. She's Vietnamese."

Another round of keening erupts from the room. It is heartbreaking in its torment. I move past Lorna into the room and close the door behind me. On the bed lies an emaciated old man, his eyes still open, staring sightlessly and endlessly past the ceiling; his toothless mouth is open, a yawning chasm evoking either awe or sheer terror at having crossed the threshold so recently. Flung across his body is the slight figure of a very young Asian woman dressed in a long-sleeved white blouse, black pants, and slippers. She could not be older than her mid-twenties. Certainly she looks more like she should be the old man's granddaughter, not his wife. She is clutching mightily at his bed sheets as she anguishes her loss.

"Mrs. McPherson?" I ask gently as I move in closer.

She lifts her head and looks at me through tear-stained eyes, but merely returns her attention back to her husband's body. Her shrieking wails echo and fill up the room with something dense and concrete. It is grief.

I reach over and close the dead man's eyes and rest my hand on her shoulder while she keens and keens. I realize that the man probably did function more like a father to her than a husband. And that she is probably lost here without any other family. As she shakes the bed with her wails, I wonder what will become of her.

Lorna softly pads into the room. "Well?" she asks expectantly. I am thinking she expects me to somehow produce a magic wand to fix this situation, to make it more palatable for everyone involved. The patient, the wife, the staff, the other patients on the unit. I don't have any such magic wand.

I look up at her and all I can say is, "Let's just keep the door closed and stay with her, Lorna."

"But what about the other patients?"

"They don't know they are in a hospital where people can die from their cancers?"

She looks at me steadily and sees that I really don't have a magic trick in my bag for this.

"There is nothing to do about this, Lorna. This is something to *be* with, not *do* with."

She gradually nods her head, seems to relax, and takes a seat next to the wife on the bed. She puts a hand on Mrs. McPherson's shoulder as the young widow continues to rock and wail over her husband's corpse.

"She doesn't even speak English," Lorna muses. Then she looks up at me. "You go. I'll stay with her. And go ahead and shut the door when you leave."

I rub her cheek in solidarity and back out of the room slowly. As with earlier in the day, I can't help but sense that Mr. McPherson is still floating around here, hardly able to contain his joy that he is no longer constrained by the vessel his widow is clinging to so fiercely. I wish that I could share that sentiment with her, but I know that even if I could, it would not mitigate the righteous grief she is laying claim to right now.

27

SEE NO EVIL

As I walk down the hallway, I run into Jerry as he packs his arms full of dressing change materials.

"Got enough four by fours there, Jer?" I ask, as several packages roll to the floor. I stoop to retrieve them and start packing the extras into an unused bath basin.

He nods in the direction of the adjacent room. "These are for Mike Lang's fistula."

I nod and immediately understand. Mike is an unassuming, single, middle-aged man whose widowed mother dotes on him still. The staff has adopted both of them, but tends to be protective of Mrs. Lang the most. She has become the Aunt Bea of the unit. She is also convinced that her son, who has been in treatment on and off for years, is going to be cured. He may be healed, I think to myself, but it is unlikely his body will ever be cured.

"You need an extra hand in there?" I ask.

"Sure—come on in. I never refuse help," Jerry grins back at me boyishly.

Our arms full of dressing change kits, we back-end into the room, bumping the door open. Mrs. Lang is sitting in the corner, her cane resting on the arm of the chair. Her silver white hair is done up in a coifed bun that most likely has been her only hairstyle for the last 30 years. She is dressed formally in an olive green tweed suit with a tailored blouse, full hose, and those wonderful old lady shoes my grandmother always wore. She looks over the rims of her eyeglasses from the book she is reading and smiles sweetly at us.

"Oh look, Mike, who's come to check on us." She closes her book, lays it aside, and politely gives us her undivided attention.

Jerry dumps the dressing change materials on the bedside table and then looks up at her with a smile, "Hi there, Mrs. L. Come to change Mike's dressing."

"I'm glad it's you, Jerry. You have such a wonderful way with Mike."

Mike, lying in the bed, starts rolling automatically over on his side.

"Mike, did you want to bolus yourself first with some pain medicine before you start moving around so much?" I ask, noticing his grimace.

"That's a good idea," he says and pushes the PCA button, the ping confirming that the pain medication is en route.

"How are you doin'?" he asks as I sit down next to him.

"Thought I'd come by and help Jerry. But it's just really an excuse to catch up with you."

He smiles at me as he settles into the dressing change position for the thousandth time. Mike has a hole in his back about the size of a large grapefruit. Inside the hole, the contents of his bowel drip into the cavity of his abdomen because a stubborn fistula refuses to heal. A real infection risk if there ever was one. He has had so much radiation and chemotherapy that he is a poor surgical risk; his tissues just disintegrate like melted butter when handled. It must be a gruesome prospect to face the future. I can't imagine how much pain he must be in from this. And we know the dressing changes are no picnic.

"Let me know, Jerry, when you're ready, and I'll come around the other side to help."

"No problem," Jerry responds as he begins setting up the supplies as he is going to need them.

"So, Mike, what's the latest?" I ask.

"I've been trying to convince them to discharge me. Other than the wound care, I don't think there is much more that can be done for me here."

Mrs. Lang won't hear of it. "Nonsense, Mike. Don't talk like that. How are you going to get well, thinking like that?"

Mike looks at me and says, very softly, "What the hell am I going to do with my mother?" He shakes his head as if her denial is just another cross for him to bear. Insult added to injury. I know he has tried to talk her out of cheerleading him before, but it only entrenches her further into her unrealistic hope that somehow everything will be all right and her son will go home a cured man. He must be so lonely in all this. At a time when it would be healing to be able to confide in his mother about his hopes and fears, it is her that he must take care of.

I look over Mike's body to where Jerry is all set up, and he gives me a meaningful look, which is neutral enough for Mrs. Lang to be unable to read.

"Can you cut me some tape over here?" Jerry asks.

"Sure, Jer." I squeeze Mike's shoulder and join Jerry on the opposite side of the bed.

Mrs. Lang resumes reading her book facing her bedfast son. As Jerry begins pulling off the top dressing, I am once again amazed that a living human being can have a hole this large in his body. Using sterile tweezers, Jerry begins to remove the packing from Mike's back. Mike flinches a bit.

"Sorry there, Mike," Jerry apologizes. "I'll try to go easy on you. If you need more pain medicine, I can override the pump."

"No, I'm all right," Mike says patiently.

Jerry continues. As the packing unwinds out of the hole, thick gobs of mucus, bloody tissue, and even fecal matter discharge out of his back. It is as if we are watching Mike's body liquefy from the inside out. I realize that both Jerry and I have automatically switched to mouth-breathing as the stench is powerful enough to knock us off our feet. I think of how it is for Mike to be smelling the inside of his decaying body.

"How you doin', partner?" Jerry asks.

"I'm hanging in there," Mike responds. Ever-so-patient, Mike.

"I'm sure it must be looking better now, dear," Mrs. Lang opines. "They've been working on closing this hole for such a long time."

Mike sighs heavily on the bed and hits the PCA button, but it's not time yet.

"I can get that for you, Mike," says Jerry, and reaches over to manually override the pump.

"Actually," I say, noticing the timing of Mike's efforts to bolus himself with more pain medication coming at the same time as his mother's remark, "I wonder, Mrs. Lang, when was the last time you saw Mike's wound?"

"Oh, dear, I've never seen his wound. Usually the nurses ask me to leave the room during dressing changes. Only Jerry lets me stay in here while he's working on Mike."

I look at Jerry intentionally and say, "Well, I wonder if it isn't about time for you to come over here and see what Mike's wound is looking like these days."

Jerry gives me a look. This is not usual protocol. Indeed, for any unpleasant or uncomfortable procedures, we ask family members to leave the room so as not to distress them too much. But Mike is so distressed about his mother's refusal to accept the reality of his condition that it may be time to break with protocol.

"What do you say, Mike?" I ask. "Would that be all right with you?"

I can't see Mike's face from where I am standing behind him as I assist Jerry, but he immediately and without hesitation says, "Okay by me."

Mrs. Lang looks a little confused. "Are you sure, dear?" she asks her son.

"Sure, Mom. I think it would be a really good idea for you to see it." It seems to me that Mike intuitively understands my invitation to his mother and that he is tacitly agreeing to this bid to help her come to terms with the severity of his condition.

"Well, all right, dear, if you want me to." She lays aside her book and rocks to a standing position, cane in hand, making her way slowly around the bed to where Jerry is continuing to unpack Mike's wound. About the time she joins us, a fairly large splinter of bony material pops out of the wound with the packing. This is not lost on her.

"Oh, Mikey," she gasps, her freed hand covering her mouth. She almost looks like she is going to vomit when she sees the residue of her son's body lying on the chux pad on the bed. "Oh, Mikey!" And she turns and leaves the room as quickly as someone on a cane possibly can.

"You got this, Jerry?" I ask.

He nods and says, "You better get out there."

"Is my mother okay?" Mike asks, alarmed.

"I think she got your message finally, Mike," is all Jerry says as he begins to irrigate the wound.

Mike lets out a big sigh and surrenders visibly to the bed.

I leave them to it and find Mrs. Lang making her way down the hallway. She is obviously disturbed.

"Why did you make me see that?" she asks as I catch up to her. "I had no idea."

"Exactly, Mrs. Lang. I just wanted you to understand what Mike is up against every time you ask him to keep on fighting."

"I'm very upset right now. I don't want to talk about it."

"I can see that. I know you might be very upset with me, but I'd like to talk to you about this the next time I see you. It is a shock to see it up close. I'm sorry, but you didn't appear to understand the severity of Mike's condition. This seemed one way to help close the gap between where he is and where you are."

"I really don't want to talk about it any more right now." And with that she enters the rest room, leaving me outside in the hallway.

I am, of course, ambivalent about my course of action. Have I been too harsh in my efforts to advocate on Mike's behalf? Could I have done this another way? I know I will be following up with her tomorrow, so it isn't over. Sometimes the work I do does not fit the stereotype of the touchy feely caregiver. Sometimes the work is that of tough love, and as such, it is a tough sell. Even to me. I blow her a metaphorical kiss through the restroom door when the pager goes off.

28

Does Allah Punish Vanity?

"This is Patrice." I say, wandering down the hallway just in case Mrs. Lang comes out. I don't want her to think I'm waiting outside the restroom to ambush her.

"Yes, I don't know if I'm talking to the right person or not. This is Nancy up in General Surgery next door. Is this the psych CNS?"

"Yes, what can I do for you, Nancy?" This is the second time today I'm being called by someone not in my own hospital. Is there a run going on?

"This is probably an unusual request, but we have a patient up here, and we could use some help."

"Okay, what seems to be the problem?"

"Well, she's had a mastectomy."

"If she's had a mastectomy, why isn't she with us?" I ask, surprised.

"Well, that's the thing. She had a gastric bypass and developed a fistula between her stomach and her chest wall that became so extensive she had to have her breast removed."

I let out a long whistle despite myself.

"Yeah, it's all that. And more," Nancy says. "Can you come by to see her?"

"I'm on my way if you can tell me where you are."

Whenever I think I've heard them all, I hear a new one.

Nancy is waiting for me outside the nurse's station and smiles at me warmly as she shows me to a corner where we can sit and talk, away from the flurry of activity.

"This is Keisha Mohammed, a 29-year-old patient of Dr. Garth's. Keisha, who is only five foot three, weighed about 320 pounds. She decided to have a gastric bypass procedure done and spent all of last year going through the pre-certification process and patient education program to qualify. She had the procedure and was doing well, but little by little, she began to notice changes in her left breast. Asymmetry, discoloration, things like that. By the time they took a look at her, they ended up deciding on mastectomy because the lumpectomy they thought they could originally do was going to be so mutilating that it would be better to consider mastectomy with eventual reconstruction."

"Holy smokes," I say. "This is a new one on me."

"On all of us," Nancy agrees, sipping from a cup of cold coffee. "Anyway, she is estranged from her husband, and she is Muslim. So this is posing a lot of difficulties for her."

"I guess so," I say. "Does she know to expect me?"

She nods. "Yes. Actually, I asked her first before I called you. Room 822 to your right."

And with that, I am on my way down the hall. I knock on her door and enter.

"Keisha Mohammed?"

"Yes." The beautiful, large woman in bed looks up at me. She has a mane of curly dark hair that cascades over an explosively colorful caftan. She is fully made up and coifed, and her fingernails are painted to perfection. Whatever I was expecting, it isn't this.

I introduce myself, and she tells me in precise diction that she has been expecting me and to please take a seat. I tell her what Nancy has already told me.

"So what has been the hardest part of this entire experience?" I ask her, cutting to the chase.

"I am feeling guilty about my mastectomy," she replies, continuing to rub lotion very carefully up her arms and around her hands as she speaks.

"How so?" I ask, settling in, crossing my legs.

"If I had not been so vain, I would still have my whole body. It was Allah's way of punishing me."

"Can you help me understand?"

She continues with the lotion, this time moving to her feet, rather sensuously lathering them as she talks.

"I did not want my husband looking at other women."

"And having the gastric bypass would ensure that?"

She nods. "I knew I was overweight, and to a point, my husband enjoyed me that way. You see, he didn't like other men looking at me either. But it got to a certain point that I became so overweight, I could not lose any of it. And then my husband became somewhat disinterested in me, and I thought I needed to do something more drastic."

She could be talking about the weather but for the erotic movement of her fingers, up and down her legs. The self-massage is almost mesmerizing to watch. I feel like a voyeur, and after a time, find myself relaxing simply from being witness to it. She caps the tube of massage lotion, the scent wafting into the air as she fluffs out the bed linens and re-settles herself. Like a queen, I think.

"And so now, Allah is showing me the error of my ways. I am being punished for being so vain."

"Is Allah really so vindictive that you would be punished for this?"

"Yes," she says quite simply.

"Is this what your husband believes as well?"

"As you probably see, I am an African-American. I con-verted to Islam when I met my husband. He came to this country from Africa. But you see, African men expect their women to serve them, and he does not understand that American women are not like that. We have had a lot of trouble at home. I have tried hard to come around to his point of view, but I do have my limits."

"So, this is difficult now because you have adopted the religion of your husband, but now you and your husband are . . . ?"

"Let us say, we are separated right now," she says care-fully, as she pulls out a nail file, and begins to work on her fingernails.

"And so, I am wondering if you will ever be able to forgive yourself if you believe that Allah finds you unforgivable."

"Oh, I don't believe that Allah finds me unforgivable. But I do believe that I am definitely being punished for my transgression."

"Would it help to speak to a mullah about this?" I ask.

"Oh, yes, my mullah is the one who is teaching me through this experience."

I don't know enough about the Koran to understand the finer workings of her thinking.

"I am not here to impose my beliefs upon you," I say, treading carefully, "but I cannot help but feel sad that you feel you are being punished by a vengeful God who could be more available to you if you believed God was a source of compassion and forgiveness."

"You misunderstand me, Ms. Rancour. I am not saying that my God is not compassionate. However, God does expect obedience. And I disobeyed."

She puts down her nail file and stares straight at me. "You know, I was raised a Baptist, so I know where you are coming from. But that Baptist God could also smite you if you disobeyed."

"I certainly am not here to argue the finer points of how many angels can dance on the head of a pin. I only hope you can find it in your own heart to forgive yourself for whatever you believe you have done. I think it would be very healing for you right now. Truly."

"I appreciate that you are trying to help me, but really, I am fine. Really." She goes back to manicuring her nails.

I feel like I have been dismissed. I pull out a card from my overstuffed pocket and hand it to her.

"If you would ever like to talk again. About anything. Please do call me. I'd like to understand more how this is for you."

She takes the card, examines it carefully, slides it onto the bedside table, and offers me her hand to shake as she looks up at me.

"Thank you so much for your time," she says with elegance. "I will think about what you have said."

"It was a pleasure meeting you," I reply as I take her hand. I notice, as I close the door behind me, that she is once again intent on her manicure. Well, this has been a wild ride, I think. I doubt she will call me back. I write up the consult and slip it onto the top of her chart for Nancy who is nowhere to be seen in the nurse's station.

And that's when the pager goes off again.

29

TRYING TO GET TO HEAVEN

It's Nadine from Pain Service again. "We have a situation here and wondered if you could help."

"Okay, what's up?"

"We've been seeing Beverly Jackson, a 34-year-old uterine cancer patient of Dr. Ramirez, for pain control for the past five days. I think she is pretty well understanding that she is end-stage and would like to talk to someone about it. Can you help out?"

"Sure, I'm on my way," I reply. I spring down the stairs to the sky-bridge that gets me back into my own hospital again. As I enter the room where Nadine is finishing up with the patient, an older woman and a younger man follow me in. They slide off their coats, and approach both Nadine and me at the bedside as Nadine is introducing me to Beverly.

"And you are?" the older woman asks me as Nadine leaves the room. The younger man towering over her must be her son. His fingers dazzle with gold rings.

"Mama, she's here to talk to me about my options," Beverly says as she repositions herself with effort on the bed.

Her mother immediately takes a protective, defensive stance. "What kind of options?"

"I just want to hear about my choices if I decide I don't want any more chemotherapy."

"Nonsense," her mother glowers. "Where's your fight, girl? You have to keep a positive attitude."

"Mama, this is my decision, not yours," Beverly sighs as she attempts a reposition in the bed. "Please don't do this." She looks straight at me and says with an equal amount of determination, "Please, go on."

Beverly's mother's cold stare could drop me dead on the spot. Her brother interrupts her.

"Now, come on B, don't be doin' that stuff. You're going to make out okay."

"I want to hear what she has to say," Beverly repeats, looking straight at me.

Considering the amount of overt hostility in the room, I know I am not going to make much headway with Beverly. I walked into a family with enough baggage on the subject to fill all the closets on the unit. And then some.

"Bev, I have some literature in my office I could drop off for you to look over first, and then we could talk more about it later," I decide. "But right now, I see that there is a fairly large difference of opinion about your treatment here. Do you all want to talk about it?"

Bev's brother slams his fist down on the bedside table and sends some paper cups full of water flying. Bev does not react to his threat. She must be used to it. Her mother is glowering at me. I once again leave a card at the bedside table with the offer that if they change their minds, they can certainly get in touch with me.

"What do you want me to do, Beverly? I can stay or leave right now." Now that I have met her brother, I am not sure if his behavior puts her at risk somehow.

"We're leaving," her mother hisses, as the brother follows her out the door.

Beverly takes a deep breath and looks over at me. "Now you know what I'm up against," she says.

"They sure are pouring on the pressure. Must be hard to make a decision."

"No actually, it is not hard. It is my decision. I just wish they could be a part of it is all." She yawns deeply. "You know, that just exhausted me. Do you mind dropping over those brochures and coming back another time when they won't be here? I've got to make my plans. I'm just so tired right now."

"No problem. I'll make sure you have them before I leave work today," I say, squeezing her shoulder. Her eyes are already closing.

Nadine is in the nurse's station charting as I pass by.

"Done so soon?" she looks up, surprised.

I explain what happened as I make a note to drop off the literature to Beverly.

She briefly shakes her head, blowing a strand of graying hair up from her forehead.

The set to her mouth is firmly drawn.

"Crazy, no?" she asks, more to herself than to me.

"What do you mean?" I pull up the chair next to her as she cradles her head in the hand holding the pen.

"Oh, I don't know. This place. What being in a place like this does to people."

"How do you mean?"

She puts the pen down and closes the chart. "Oh, I'm just thinking about what happened on the other pod this morning with a patient we were following." She looks thoughtful, like she'd like to talk, but I see her glance at her watch.

"I'm all ears," I say as if I've already settled in. I'm again reminded of that old maxim that in the hearing is the learning, but in the telling is the healing. Patients aren't the only ones in need of healing.

"We've been following a patient from BMT who has been deteriorating rather steadily. Too many complications. This past week had been particularly bad for her."

"Had been?"

She nods. "This morning her parents came in, thinking that a procedure they had talked about last night with one of the surgeons was going to save the day for her. But there was a question about the date being—"propitious"—I think that was the word they used."

"Let me guess. Were they East Indian?"

"She nods." You know them?"

"No, I just ran into them in the elevators a little while ago. What happened?"

"They are such a wonderful family. This was their only daughter. Her name was Chandani."

"Was?"

"Let me finish," she sighs.

"Anyway, she threw a clot this morning and was made a DNR. The parents asked the attending to be able to place their daughter on the floor. As Hindus, they want to be as close to the ground as possible when they die."

"What happened?"

"The attending refused. Told them it would be an infection risk. That we have infection control policies."

"You have got to be kidding. We're worrying about an infection at the time of death? Like we couldn't put her on a clean blanket on the floor?"

"Sister, you are singing to the choir."

"So, what happened?"

"We waited for the attending to leave the unit. And then we put Chandani on a clean blanket on the floor." We both look at each other solemnly. "And that's when Chandani went to heaven," Nadine finished.

I think about the couple from the elevator. So filled with hope on the way up to see their only daughter. I think of them looking for a propitious date. I think of them begging us to place her on the floor so that she can be close to the earth when she dies.

My heart fills up.

Nadine and I give each other sad smiles. A rich knowing passes between us. She places a hand on my shoulder as she rises.

"I have to get to the treatment room," she whispers.

I nod as the pager goes off again.

30

This Old Man Can't Take Much More of This

"Hi, it's Patrice," I reply.

It's Carla on 7. "It's Mr. Cardoza in 42. I know you've been working with him and his family. He seems really despondent today. I couldn't squeeze a smile out of him if my life depended on it."

Mr. Cardoza has undergone a radical neck dissection and has had his voice box removed. His only daughter lives out of town, and his wife is newly diagnosed with Alzheimer's. He breathes through a hole in his neck and reminds me of that Harlan Ellison science fiction short story called "I Have No Mouth, and I Must Scream."

"Well," I muse, "I don't think he has much to smile about right now."

Carla agrees. "Well, just thought you'd like to keep your finger on that pulse."

"I appreciate it, Carla. I'll be up in a minute."

When I enter the room, Mr. Cardoza is in bed, looking out the window. His attentive daughter and unfortunate wife are sitting silently on the other side of the room. They look up at me expectantly.

"Mrs. Cardoza, Lisa." I turn toward Mr. Cardoza, but he doesn't look back at me. I move in closer and say gently, "Carla tells me you've been feeling really blue today. Care to talk about it?" Of course, talking is just a euphemism with Mr. Cardoza.

He coughs and a mucus plug is dislodged from his trach tube. He swabs at it, picking up a white board and magic marker from the bed, removing whatever was written on it before with a paper towel. He writes with a kind of shorthand, like someone who has wearied of having to communicate by hand all the time. He hands it over to me and looks back out the window.

Even his penmanship looks despairing. He has written, "this old man can't take much more of this."

I glance over at him. He is not expecting much. I turn it over to show it to his wife and daughter. They both lower their eyes. His wife turns away, stifling a quiet cry.

"Can we talk about this?" I ask quietly.

Lisa approaches her father's bed. "Dad? Is this the way you really feel?"

He does not turn toward her. I understand then how really angry he is that all of this is unfolding as it is. And how unable he is to really express it. After all, he has been robbed of a voice. He nods imperceptibly.

Lisa turns to her mother. "Mom, we really need to talk this through."

Her mother is unable to turn around and just puts up a hand to stop her daughter. I wait several moments to give

Mrs. Cardoza a chance to regroup, and then I approach her slowly.

"It's too much to face all at once, isn't it, Mrs. Cardoza?" I say to her gently. She turns around and looks at me, nodding as the tears flow silently down her cheeks.

"I am so sorry for your pain," I say. "All of it," I add, alluding to her new Alzheimer's diagnosis.

She nods as she wipes her face. I think, God love her, as she works to reclaim her dignity in front of me. She approaches her husband's bed from the window side so that he is forced to deal with her and doesn't turn away. She reaches out a tentative hand and sweeps a few long strands of "comb-over" white hair wisps back from his face. He looks at her for the longest time, and takes her hand, pressing it against his silent lips, then places her hand on his heart.

The better part of valor sometimes lies in learning when to bow out. I gesture to Lisa that I am going to leave as I do not want to intrude into whatever is going to happen here. She nods and quietly takes a seat in the corner. She indicates she will call me later. I give her a complicit smile and close the door behind me.

And, the pager goes off. It's Marvelle.

31

I'D RATHER BE FISHIN'

"It's Mrs. Whitacker calling for you. She says she's left you a message on your office phone, but you haven't returned it yet."

"I haven't been able to get back to my office all day, Marvelle. But you can transfer it here to the station on 7. I'll pick it up here. Thanks."

I make my way to the nurse's station where a line is already ringing where no one is sitting.

The Whitacker's have been through it. An older middle-aged couple, they had been living in the foothills of the mountains. When I first met Ernie, he was being prepped for a hemipelvectomy. This is not just a leg amputation. This is an amputation that removes the entire side of a hip on down. He had worked hard to save the leg that was being invaded by an osteosarcoma, but the tumor was just too aggressive.

I was with him in the SICU as he was waking up after surgery. A nurse had come in to do an assessment, and had asked him off-handedly how much he weighed. He started to reply, "Two hundred . . ." and then looked at me in some confusion. "How the hell am I supposed to know how much I weigh now?"

Later, I had hooked Ernie up with John, someone who had already been through similar surgery. I had wanted to make sure he could see there was life after hemipelvectomy. I'll never forget the look on his face when a tissue box had tipped over to the floor, and John had reached over in one fell swoop, without using a cane or walker, to retrieve it. When he replaced it on Ernie's over-the-bed table, he caught the surprise on his face, and simply muttered, "Hey brother, it's a cakewalk."

But it wasn't. A week later, during the course of Ernie's work with physical therapy, the medical oncologists had shared with him that the sarcoma had metastasized to his lungs which would require chemotherapy. I remember his hang-dog look at me. "If I'd known that, I would've never had this damn surgery," he'd said.

I remember looking at him thoughtfully at the time. "Well, Ernie, if you weren't here receiving chemotherapy, where would you rather be?"

Without skipping a beat, Ernie replied, "Well, I'd be fishin' down at the lake back home."

We talked further a bit about the decisions he was facing, and I promised him I'd return the next day. When I made rounds the next morning, the bed was occupied by someone else, usually not a good sign.

"What happened to Ernie Whitacker?" I asked the unit secretary.

She fished something out of a file drawer as she answered. "He decided to leave last night."

"Did he mention why?"

She shrugged, "Said he'd rather be fishing."

I had smiled to myself, picturing him on his boat at this very moment, throwing out a line. Several months later, we had learned that he had died. But at least he'd gone out on his own terms. That was quite some time ago already, come to think of it.

I pick up the phone. "Florence?"

"Is this Patrice?" the voice, with a slight drawl to it asks.

"Yes."

"Thank God. Yes, it's me. I been tryin' to reach you all day. Where you been?"

"I'm sorry, Florence. What can I do for you?"

"Well, it's about Ernie. I think he's still here."

"How do you mean, Florence?"

"Ever since Ernie died, there's been a black presence in the house. It's been tryin' to get rid of me." She speaks in hushed tones, as if afraid she will be overheard.

"A black presence? Can you describe it in more detail, Florence?"

"Well, it's not a person, if that's what you're thinkin.' It's more like a feelin' I git when I'm in the house. It feels like a big black cloud trying to throw me outta my own home."

"What makes you think it's Ernie?"

"Well, it started happenin' right after Ernie left me. What else could it be?"

"Have you ever had this happen to you before, Florence? A feeling of a big black cloud?"

A long silence. "Well, come to think of it, when my mama died about twenty years ago, she visited me that way, too."

"Florence, I really don't think it was your mother. And I don't think this is Ernie. I think you're having a grief reaction. You miss Ernie. Like you missed your mother."

"No, I'm not kidding. This feels real personal, Patrice. It's tryin' to get rid of me. I swear. It chases me from room to room."

"Florence, have you told anyone down there about this?"

"What, are you crazy? They'd have me locked up for sure."

"You haven't told anyone in your family?"

"Nope, and I ain't gonna either."

"What about your family doctor?"

"He'd just send me off to one of those funny doctors, don't ya know."

"What about your pastor?"

"I did tell him, but he already come over to bless the house and exorcise whatever it is. 'Cept it's still here." She stops talking suddenly and is breathing very hard.

"Florence, what is it?"

"It just come in the room. It knows I'm talkin' about it."

I am now understanding this may be more than just a complicated bereavement. In the absence of her willingness to ask anybody local for help, I press her.

196

"What's it like being with it?" I ask.

"I'm scared to death," she says, whispering over the phone. I can hear her cupping the receiver.

"Tell it how you're feeling, and ask it what it wants from you that it's been hanging around you so much. Listen to what it says, and then tell me."

"You want me to talk to it? Are you outta your mind?"

"No, go ahead, Florence. Let's figure this out. Now. While we're together on the phone. The chances of my coming down there in person are pretty slim."

I can tell she's sorry she called, but she doesn't hang up the phone either. I hear her talking in the background. And then she is back on the line.

"It says it wants me to leave."

"Ask it why."

I hear her echo the question. "Because it says I need to be with Ernie."

"Ask it what it means by that."

More talking. "It says Ernie wants me to get out to the lake more." The tone of her voice is starting to shift more from fear to curiosity.

"So it's not Ernie, then."

"I guess not," she says in a quiet voice. "Well, I'm glad 'bout that at least."

On a hunch, I say, "Ask it if you can talk directly to Ernie."

"Okay." I can tell she'd rather be talking to anybody but the big black cloud.

"What's happening?"

"Nothing yet."

"Call Ernie's name."

She does. And then there's a pause and a slight gasp of air.

"Ernie's here," she says breathlessly.

"Where's the cloud?"

"It disappeared."

"Can you see Ernie?"

"No, more like I can feel him here with me." Her voice sounds soothed and surprised at the same time.

"Ask Ernie what he wants."

A pause. "Like the cloud said before, he wants me to get out more."

"Sounds like he's worried about you."

Another pause. "He says he's never left me. That I should be gettin' on with my life, because he's with me everywhere I go. That I should leave the house more."

"So you haven't been leaving the house much?"

"No, because this is where I feel closest to him."

"It sounds like he wants you to know that it doesn't matter where you are. That he's never going to leave you."

"Yeah," she says skeptically. "That's what it sounds like."

"So how long have you been cooped up in the house, Florence? Ever since Ernie passed?"

"Pretty much," she muses.

"Well that's been months and months, hasn't it?" I ask.

"Well, yeah, I guess."

"You know, Florence, that's not healthy for you."

"I know. My kids have been on me 'bout it, but it's just been so hard here without Ernie." She suddenly starts weeping. "You don't know what it's like. Me an' him have been together ever since we was sixteen."

I listen to her choking on the other end of the line.

"Florence, would you give me permission to call your doctor and talk to him about what's been going on?"

"I don't want him to think I need a nut house," she says defensively.

"I promise that is not how I will describe it," I promise.

"What're you gonna say to him?"

"I'm going to tell him you've been having trouble ever since Ernie died. That you have had a bad grief reaction and that you've been having trouble getting back into the swing of things. Florence, you may be depressed, and he can help you find someone to talk to, perhaps even give you some medicine to help with this. It will not always feel this way, Florence."

She reluctantly agrees and gives me her doctor's name and phone number. I ask her to call him first to give him permission to speak with me.

"What'll I do about Ernie and the black cloud?"

"Well, I'm thinking the black cloud won't be bothering you any more. Now that you can speak with Ernie directly. Why don't you ask him if that will be okay with him?"

She does. "He says it's okay with him." I hear more talking on the other end of the line. "He also says to thank you and to let you know the fishin's fine, whatever that means."

I can't help but smile to myself. "Tell Ernie I'm glad to hear it. Oh, and Florence, I'll be calling you in a couple of days to check up on you, okay?"

"Okay," she says, a little sheepishly. "I hope I'm not gonna be sorry about callin' you up there."

"Florence, please have a little faith. Okay?"

"Okay. I'll talk to you in a couple a days." And she hangs up.

I think of Florence all alone in that little house up in the hills. I'm hoping her doctor will be receptive to my phone call and that we will be able to find some help for her in a town where I don't know a soul and people talk. I write a note to myself in my little black book just as the pager goes off.

FAMILY MATTERS

"Hi, it's Paula in the MICU."

"What can I do for you, Paula?"

"It's a patient we have here, a Mr. Walter King. His lymphoma has been refractory to all treatment, and when he became unresponsive, his family asked he be put on life support here. He's been with us now for more than three weeks with no change, and his family insists he remain here until he recovers. The docs believe that he will not recover, but the family is pretty insistent. We were hoping you could come over to work with the family."

"So, no living will or durable power of attorney identified, no doubt." It was more of a statement than a question. "How do we let people get to this point, and not start working with them on advance directives when they still can?"

"You're singing to the choir," Paula says. "Quite frankly, we're dead in the water here. The family is formidable."

"I get the picture. Is the family over there now?"

"Yup."

"Okay, but I left my magic wand at home today. Just so you know."

Her smile is almost audible over the phone. "I hear you."

Walter King is a handsome elderly black man who is essentially in a coma. Even in his present condition, it is easy to see that this man is the rock of his large family. They are distributed around his bed like courtiers around the throne. There is a palpable feeling of filial devotion here.

I introduce myself, and they introduce themselves to me. Each of them is accomplished professionally or artistically. A pharmacist. A professional dancer. A successful entrepreneur. A college professor. A journalist. They introduce their mother, an elegant woman with close cropped hair, spare makeup, and understated jewelry, who stands by the head of her husband's bed. She is the picture of dignity.

"I understand that Mr. King has been sick a long time," I begin.

"He stood by each of us when we were sick," responds the dancer. She is the spitting image of her mother, lithe and dressed simply, yet with a stylish grace. The remark is edged in a bit of guardedness, almost as if they are already primed to defend the current decision to stay the course, no matter what.

Her brothers and sister nod their heads, and their attention is drawn back to their father in the bed.

"It must be hard to watch your father go through this. He looks like he must have been a very strong person."

"That is why we are trying to give him a chance," responds the pharmacist. "He has come through worse than this before. With God's grace, he will come through this as well."

I try again. "Had you ever had any discussions with him prior to this when he shared with you what he might have wanted if ever faced with this situation?"

His wife looks at me levelly. "Where there is breath, there is life. My husband believed this and taught our children to believe this as well. It is a deeply held religious conviction that we all hold."

A brick wall. I can see why the intensivist is trying to call in whatever cavalry she can find in order to begin the difficult work of transitioning this family from curative treatment goals to the more palliative treatment goals of comfort care.

I say nothing for a few moments. I feel cowed by their shared denial, and their staunch belief that this man is so strong that he is even above dying. I need to tread softly here so that I don't offend them, and create even more entrenchment.

I have been thinking about this so hard that I miss the journalist studying me. Paula comes in to recalibrate an IV drip and reprogram some of the equipment.

The journalist asks Paula, "Did you send her in here to deal with us?" He nods his head in my direction.

"Actually," Paula smiles, "We asked her to come in for us."

The journalist looks puzzled at this, but doesn't say anything.

The entrepreneur says, "You know, you will all be surprised when my father opens his eyes again. But we won't be. God is taking care of him."

Paula gives me a camouflaged, if exasperated eye roll, and I try to seize this opening as an opportunity.

"Well, Mr. King, no matter what happens, I believe God is taking care of your father."

The journalist hears this as me laying down a gauntlet, and so rises to the occasion to meet it. "Because God is taking care of him, he will recover."

And that is when I understand that pushing further will accomplish nothing here. I look at the rise and fall of Mr. King's chest as the ventilator continues to push in the oxygen. I wonder if he can hear what is going on. I wonder if he could weigh in, what would he say. To all of us. I frankly have no idea.

I tell them that it was an honor to meet them and that I will look in on them from time to time if that is all right. They answer diplomatically by keeping their attention on Mr. King lying there in the bed. I withdraw.

I sit down next to Paula in the nurse's station. She glances over at me.

"See what I mean?" she says. "They're tough."

"Either that, or he's very lucky to have them advocating for him like that."

"Lucky only if he recovers tomorrow. Not so lucky if he is doomed to go on like this for months and months and months."

I nod in agreement.

"Well, since I left my crystal ball with my magic wand, I can't say. You know, their faith plays a large measure in this. Has anyone contacted their pastor?"

"I'm not sure," she says, giving it some thought. "Pastoral Care has been involved with them. I can ask them if the family has had contact with their own clergy."

"I'm thinking that if they hear this from their own clergy person, perhaps it will be more acceptable. This is really a matter of faith for them, not science. We're only a bunch of white lab coats to them."

She nods. "I'll call down to Pastoral Care, and see if they can contact the family's own pastor. Perhaps that is the way to go here. Certainly nothing we say is having any effect."

"Kind of like working with Teflon, huh?"

She grins in agreement.

"Sorry, I couldn't 'abracadabra' this for you," I say as I get up to leave.

"Well, getting in touch with the pastor is a new idea in the mix. We'll give that a try and see what happens."

"Keep me posted, will you?"

"Will do," she says as she returns to her computer charting.

33

And So It Goes

I take a deep breath and look at my watch. How did it get to be 5:30? I decide that that's all I can do for today, although so many things have been left unfinished, so many things that I had meant to get completed never got started. Oh, well, what is my work if not the interruptions between what I thought I was going to do?

I return to my closet, turn off the computer that I never touched, open the drawer to get my purse, take off the frayed lab coat that I need to replace, and hang it up. I turn off the pager for the day—the pager that functions as a portal into other people's worlds.

I have the best work in the world, I think.

I realize I am starving and that my bladder is full. I walk to the elevator and find myself mercifully alone until the door opens into the lobby, and the night's evening visitors enter. I cross the lobby, filled with people coming and going, preoccupied with their own stories, their own desperations, their own lives. I push through the revolving door and out into the sunshine. The air is fresh, swept clean with the scent of evaporating puddles. The sidewalks steam with the misting vapors.

When did the torrential downpour stop, I wonder? Where did all this sunshine come from? I notice how the light filters through the leaves, how the shadows play at my feet.

As I walk past the hospital on the way to the parking lot, I glance up to the BMT floor and spot the windows behind which I know personal hells are unfolding. People I pass on the street are clueless about what is happening up there. They have their own preoccupations, their own ruminations. I whisper a short prayer for the souls upstairs and send it on its wings.

By the time I reach my car, my day has melted off me, the sun kissing me on the top of my head.

And that is when I realize that my entire day has been my prayer.

* * * * * * * * * *

The drive home is uneventful. Thankfully. I pull up my driveway, ready to start the "second shift."

As I enter the house, a voice from another room yells out, "Hey, Mama," It's my son. I think about my friend who lost her son today as my own son's tall lanky body swings into the room. I take him into my arms and squeeze him tightly. Don't want to let him go.

"What's with you, Mama?" he says mock complaining, but I know by his smile he enjoys the bear hug.

I tell him the story of my friend's son. "Do you realize how much I love you, how much I cherish you? Do you know what would happen to me if anything happened to you?" I say, frightened, yet elated at the sheer feel of him. I bury my nose into his mop of curly hair and inhale him into me.

I hear my husband pulling into the driveway. I scrounge around in the refrigerator to pull together a meal made of leftovers from the last two nights. We eat. I make a phone call. Throw in a load of laundry.

After we eat, my son suddenly remembers that he has a big term paper due the next day. He hasn't started it yet. I go into my parental rant and rave. "What can you be thinking?!"

He admonishes me slyly, "Whatever happened to how much you cherish me, Mama?"

Much later, well into the night, the paper finally sweated over and completed, I stand at his bedside and watch as his legs twitch in response to his dreams, my breath in rhythm with his.

Watching him, I think about all the bedsides I've stood by. And all the ones yet to come.

My pager, muted and distant, bears silent witness as I ready the house and myself for bed.

And so it goes.

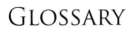

GLOSSARY

Antibiotic-Resistant Organism: A microbe that is genetically unresponsive to current antibiotic treatment, so resists eradication from the body.

Arthroscopic: Refers to a surgical technique whereby a doctor inserts a tube-like instrument into a joint to inspect, diagnose, and repair tissues. It is most commonly performed in patients with diseases of the knees or shoulders.

Attending: The patient's physician.

Bilateral Mastectomy: The surgical removal of both breasts.

BMT: Bone marrow transplant. A procedure in which the bone marrow is infused into a patient. The marrow can be from the patient or from a donor.

BMTU: Bone Marrow Transplant Unit. Where patients receive and recover from bone marrow transplants.

Bolus: A single dose of a drug administered intravenously.

Central Line: An intravenous line placed in one of the large veins in the chest (superior or inferior vena cava) for the purpose of delivering drugs (including chemotherapy) that would be too caustic to deliver by smaller veins in the arms. Since chemotherapy is given over longer periods of time, the central line access in the chest means that patients do not have to be repeatedly stuck with needles.

Charge: The charge nurse or the nurse in charge of a shift's patient and work assignments.

Code team: A highly specialized team of physicians, nurses, respiratory therapists and pharmacists who respond to all cardiopulmonary resuscitation emergencies (Code Blue) in the hospital. The cart that contains emergency drugs and equipment is referred to as the crash cart.

Colostomy: Refers to a surgical procedure whereby a portion of the large intestine is brought through the abdominal wall to carry stool out of the body.

Complementary and Alternative Medicine (CAM): A group of diverse medical and health care systems, practices, and products that are not presently considered to be part of conventional medicine. These include modalities from bioenergetics, mind-body connection practices, somatic or body-work type of practices, herbal/botanical, and supplements as well as entire systems of healing.

Cyborg: A human who has certain physiological processes aided or controlled by mechanical or electronic devices.

Dissociate: State of acute mental decompensation in which certain thoughts, emotions, sensations and/or memories are compartmenalized because they are too overwhelming for the conscious mind to integrate.

DSM-IV Revised: Diagnostic and Statistical Manuel of Mental Disorders. A handbook used throughout the United States by mental health professionals.

Durable Power of Attorney for Health Care: One of two Advance Directive documents (the other being the Living Will) which designates someone who will speak for the patient regarding his/her end-of-life care preferences when the patient is unable to do so.

Fistula: A permanent abnormal passageway between two organs in the body or between an organ and the exterior of the body.

Fugue State: A pathological amnesiac condition during which one is apparently conscious of one's actions but has no recollection of them after returning to a normal state of awareness.

Graft vs. Host Disease: An immune attack on the recipient by cells from a donor. Often seen in transplant cases in which the patient's own immune system attacks the donor tissue as a foreign body. The patient is then given drugs to suppress his or her own immune response in order for the new tissue to properly engraft.

Guided Imagery: The use of relaxation and mental visualization to improve mood and/or physical well-being.

Head and Neck Resection: The surgical removal of a diseased part or organ in the head and/or neck.

Immunosupressive drugs: Usually chemotherapy, but also other drugs, such as steroids, that result in the patient's immune system being compromised. In order for tumor cells to be killed, other normal immune system cells are unfortunately killed as well.

Implanted Pain Pump: A device that serves as a reservoir and delivery system for pain medication placed in the abdomen under the skin, from which a catheter is tunneled under the skin, inserted into the space of the spine, and connected to the pump. Medication can be delivered at constant or variable flow rates. Infection is minimized and freedom of the patient's movement is enhanced.

Living Will: One of two advance directive documents (the other being durable power of attorney for health care) that delineates the patient's end-of-life care preferences should the patient be permanently unconscious or in a persistent vegetative state.

MICU: Medical Intensive Care Unit. A critical-care unit for patients with serious medical conditions.

MRI: Magnetic Resonance Imagery: By use of strong magnets and pulses of radio waves to manipulate the natural magnetic properties in the body, this technique makes better images of organs and soft tissues than those of other scanning technologies.

Multiple Personality Disorder: Two or more distinct identities or personality states alternate in controlling the patient's consciousness and behavior. Also referred to as dissociative identity disorder.

Nasogastric Tube: A tube that is inserted through the nose and is guided into the stomach. It can be used to suction out stomach secretions or to provide tube feedings to patients who cannot swallow normally.

Ommaya Reservoir: A device implanted under the scalp that is used to deliver anticancer drugs to the cerebrospinal fluid, the fluid surrounding the brain and spinal cord.

Open and close: A slang term used by health care personnel to refer to the type of surgery done when the surgeon finds more cancer during an operation than can safely be removed and chooses instead to suture the patient with much of the cancer still present. Often these patients are referred for palliative or comfort care.

Osteosarcoma: Cancer of the bone.

PCA: Patient-Controlled Analgesia. A medication delivery system in which the patient is in charge of delivering extra doses of pain medication through a pump hooked up to an intravenous tube. The pump can be set up to deliver continuous as well as patient-initiated doses, and is often used to help titrate (determine the concentration) of the pain medication the patient requires in order to be kept comfortable.

Phantom Pain: Pain or discomfort felt by an amputee in the area of the missing limb.

Pheromones: Chemicals secreted by an organism that affect the behavior of other organisms of the same species.

Piggyack IV Solution: Usually a smaller bag of medication administered intermittently through an intravenous catheter at the same time as the main intravenous solution is infusing.

Placebo Effect: The measurable, observable, or felt improvement in health or behavior not attributable to a medication or treatment that has been administered.

Pod: A nursing unit.

Psych CNS: A psychiatric/mental health clinical nurse specialist. A nurse with a master's degree in psychiatric/mental health nursing who is board certified in that specialty by the American Nurses Credentialing Center.

Reiki: A complementary and alternative therapy based on the belief that when energy is channeled through a trained practitioner, the patient's bio-energetic field is balanced, which in turn has a healing effect upon the physical body.

Septic or Septicemia: An infection that spreads throughout the entire body by way of the circulatory system.

SICU: Surgical Intensive Care Unit. A critical-care unit for patients with serious surgical conditions.

Significance of Pain Rating Scales: A method of determining a patient's pain level. The patient is asked at regular intervals to benchmark pain on a scale of 0-10, with 0 being no pain and 10 being the worst pain imaginable. This helps health care providers to gauge the effectiveness of the patient's pain management program by increasing or decreasing pain medication dosage or by changing medications.

Split-Thickness Skin Graft: A patch of the top layer of skin that is surgically removed from one area of the body and transplanted to another area, usually to cover a wound or a burn.

Step-Down Unit: A nursing unit designed to provide care for those who need less monitoring than those in the critical care or intensive care units, but still require more monitoring than those on the medical or surgical units.

Steroid Burst: A high dose of steroids given to reduce acute inflammation and then rapidly tapered off.

Stertorous: Harsh, noisy breathing, sounding like heavy snoring, often found in comatose patients.

Tele-monitoring Devices: Electronic machines that can display different measures of the body such as blood pressure, heart rate, oxygen saturation, etc., in real time.

Discussion Questions

Discussion Questions for Health Care Professionals and Students

1. Did you identify at all with the protagonist? Why or why not? Does she allow her interactions with her patients and families to change her? In what way?

2. Do the characters seem real and believable? Can you relate to their predicaments? To what extent do they remind you of yourself or someone you know?

3. Does the protagonist allow her own views too much into the care she provides to patients? In which cases does this occur? Was it therapeutic to do so or not? Describe.

4. Were the scenes during which the protagonist had to deal with professionals of other disciplines realistic? How much inter-disciplinary conflict interferes with the effective delivery of patient care in your own work setting? How can such conflicts be resolved effectively?

5. There were a number of times when patients did not respond as the nurse had intended. When this happens, how can nurses learn from the experience?

6. How did the protagonist work in such a way as to mitigate burnout in the face of so much suffering? Are these skills teachable/learnable? How can you learn them?

7. Oftentimes in stressful work environments, health care workers have been accused of "eating their young."

In this book, does that dynamic occur? How can mentoring of the next generation be improved where you work?

8. Were you adequately prepared in your education to talk to patients and their families about death and dying? How have you learned to handle these courageous conversations that occur during critical patient care situations?

9. Inevitably, as patients and their families face the prospect of death, issues regarding spirituality surface. While pastoral care referrals are certainly encouraged, oftentimes health care workers are in excellent positions to assess and provide care designed to address the spiritual needs of their patients and families. Are you aware enough of your own ethnocentricity to avoid proselytizing your own religious views when working with others, and yet still be spiritually available to help them draw their own conclusions? If not, where can you go for help to do so?

10. The world in which we live and work has truly become multicultural and today's health care workers are expected to be able to knowledgeably serve people from different cultures. Recall the most recent experience you had with someone from a culture foreign to your own. Would you say you were culturally competent in that situation? Given additional time to think about it, what would you have done differently to have improved the process or the outcome?

11. What parts of this book were uncomfortable for you to read? Why?

12. Narrative serves many functions: it can be cathartic, educational, skill-building, mores-transferring, to name just a few. If you were to write your own non-fiction narrative, what purpose would it serve, not only for you, but also for your potential audiences?

DISCUSSION QUESTIONS FOR NON-HEALTH CARE READERS

1. When people become seriously ill, frequently it is the first time they realistically confront the prospect of their own deaths. Why do you think this is? When this has happened to you or someone you love, did any health care professional help to explore this facet of the illness? If not, would you have liked them to? Why or why not?

2. Today, pain and suffering are often "medicalized." People are often medicated for normal existential feelings such as despair and grief in the face of such suffering. Is there a place for spiritual practice within health care to deal with such suffering? If so, who should provide it?

3. Pretend you are facing a life-threatening illness. Would you choose to have your life prolonged at any cost or would you prefer to place quality of life over number of days? Do you have a living will and a durable power of attorney which describe in detail what your end of life care wishes are? If so, does anyone in your social network know about it or is it a well-kept secret? (If you don't have these advance directives documents, go to your state hospice organization's website to download the most current copies at no cost to you.)

4. When you or a loved one was treated for a serious illness, what was the one most helpful thing a health care worker said or did for you? What was the one most disturbing thing a health care worker said or did for you? Either way, did you tell them about it? Why or why not?

5. Which character did you most closely identify with in this book? Why?

6. Are you surprised by how much the protagonist allows herself to be touched by her patients and families? Is this a good thing for her professional relationships or not? Explain your point of view.

7. What specific themes did the author emphasize throughout the novel? What do you think she is trying to get across to the reader?

8. In what ways do the events in the book reveal evidence of the author's world view?

9. Did certain parts of the book make you uncomfortable? If so, why did you feel that way? Did this lead to a new understanding or awareness of some aspect of your life you might not have thought about before?

10. What in this book surprised you the most? Has reading this book changed your opinion of nurses, health care, the meaning of suffering? Death? If so, how?